THE COMPLETE ATHLETE

THE COMPLETE
ATHLETE

INTEGRATING FITNESS,
NUTRITION AND NATURAL HEALTH

John Winterdyk PhD and Karen Jensen ND

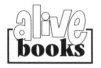

The information in this book is intended to be
used as an educational resource only.

First published in 1998 by

alive books
PO Box 80055
Burnaby, BC Canada V5H 3X1

Design by cardigan.com
Cover Photo: John P. Kelly/The Image Bank
Illustrations: Corina Messerschmidt and Rae Heald

1 3 5 7 9 10 8 6 4 2

CANADIAN CATALOGUING IN PUBLICATION DATA

Winterdyk, John
The complete athlete

Includes bibliographical references and index.
ISBN 0-920470-05-X

1. Physical education and training. 2. Athletes – Nutrition.
3. Physical fitness. I. Jensen, Karen. II. Title.

GV711.5.W56 1998   613.7'11   C98-910238-6

Printed and bound in Canada

Until one is committed

There is hesitancy, the chance to draw back, always ineffectiveness

Concerning all acts of initiative (and creation), there is one element of truth

The ignorance of which kills countless ideas and splendid plans:

That the moment one definitely commits oneself, then providence moves too.

All sorts of things occur to help one that would never have otherwise occurred

A whole stream of events issues from the decision raising in one's favor all

Manner of unforeseen incidents and meetings and material assistance which

No man could have dreamed would have come his way.

Whatever you do, or dream you can, begin it.

Boldness has genius, power and magic in it.

Begin it now.

– Goethe

Contents

Foreword

In 1982 I competed in my first Ironman triathlon. I had seen Julie Moss's dramatic crawl to the finish line of the Hawaii Ironman earlier that year and this inspired me to test the limits of my endurance and mental strength.

As my background was in swimming, I thought the transition to multi-sport racing would be easy. Much to my detriment, however, I applied archaic swim training techniques to my cycling and running. The results were not satisfactory.

During the next few years my career as a triathlete took me through many peaks and valleys. I always knew why I succeeded, but my setbacks were more of a mystery. Illness, injury and burnout always preceded a "low" period but I had difficulty anticipating when these would happen. Hindsight was my only guide to avoiding the same mistakes in the future. This learning process was a painful test of my patience, but my love of exercise and competition always carried me through.

Unfortunately, there weren't any resources in the '80s that explained in easy-to-understand terms how to avoid the pitfalls of poor training. Nor were there any good books that made it clear how to optimize my training. I was unable to find answers to my questions on diet, training techniques and injury prevention. The few books that were available were written for the experts in each field – not for multisporting athletes like me.

The kind of practical resource I always wanted – but could never find – would inspire as well as educate. At some point everybody needs a reassuring voice that says "You can reach your goals!" At last, this resource has been written and you are holding it in your hands. *The Complete Athlete* answers just about any question you might have about how to integrate your diet, training, mental attitude and overall health in your own training regime. It takes you through all the steps for implementing and maintaining a complete training program that is geared not just for performance but for overall lifestyle and health. Some of the sections answered questions I didn't even know I had! I only wish it had been around when I was racing!

– Mark Allen
Six-time Ironman Triathlon World Champion

Preface

As a young boy I loved participating in sports. My father and my Uncle "Shams" were my greatest fans and supporters. They accompanied me to the hockey rink, were there for my first bike race (age ten, I think) and taught me to play tennis and table tennis. They even gracefully endured my scathing defeats over the chessboard.

I was never forced into anything. I simply went about being just another kid discovering and enjoying the thrills of being active. In 1969, however, I had an accident that resulted in the loss of my right kidney which meant that I could no longer participate in contact sports. As I had already shown signs of becoming a promising hockey player, I recoiled in self-pity. Uncle Shams soon came to the rescue and promised he would teach me how to drive a car (strong motivation for a young man) if I agreed to take up non-contact sports. I agreed.

As I went through high school and then university, I realized how being active was critical for relieving the demands of school. While an undergraduate, I played in a competitive tennis league with modest success until a girlfriend introduced me to eating healthier! Having nothing to lose, I tried it. Well, as they say, the rest is history. My tennis improved dramatically as did my grades in school. I thought I had discovered a "big secret" – eat well, lead an active lifestyle and suddenly life is a much better passage.

Then, like so many who took up the sport of triathlon in the early eighties, watching Julie Moss cross the Hawaii Ironman finish line on her hands and knees caught my attention. The following year, to everyone's surprise, I won the Canadian Ultra Triathlon (Canadian Ironman). The announcer didn't even know how to pronounce my name! While the win was exhilarating, the "road to gold" was paved with challenges. I didn't have a clue how to train, nor did anyone else, it seemed. Two weeks before the race I could not run around the block because of an overtraining injury. As fortune would have it, though, I was introduced to Dr. Larry Chan (DC, ND) who used alternative techniques to hold me together for the race. (Conventional doctors told me to wait until next year before attempting another race.) Again, another piece of the puzzle was added to my lifestyle: eat well, stay active and support health through natural means.

– John Winterdyk, April, 1998

From a young age my quest was one of a healthy, pain-free body and inner peace. I was an active swimmer, runner, skier, hiker and cyclist. During a time in my life when I was training for the Canadian Sky Diving Team, I had an injury to my back. I was told by the medical experts that I would be in a wheelchair by the time I was thirty-five (I was twenty-four at the time). I have a very determined streak and refused to accept this diagnosis. I turned to the doctor and said, "Thank you for your opinion." and began trying to find relief from my unrelenting back pain. This began a long journey and along the way I came in contact with many alternative therapies such as naturopathic medicine and chiropractic.

As the years passed I learned many things, the most important being that life presents "learning opportunities" that are often disguised as physical, mental or emotional pain. It is up to us to chose how to embrace these opportunities so that we learn and grow from them.

Then, fourteen years ago, came another major turning point that really made me look at what I needed to do with my life. I was engaged to be married and had left the comfort of a secure job and familiar friends and family, and moved my three children to commit to our new life. While we were up skiing, my fiancé was killed in an avalanche. Without going into detail about what went through me when this happened, I was now faced with a huge question: "Now what?" Once the shock had settled somewhat, I started looking at my life and asked myself, "Other than my children, what do I really love and have a passion for?"

Since my life had revolved around health at all levels, I decided to pursue a degree in naturopathic medicine. The road seemed so long, but before I knew it, there I was, a naturopathic physician! I had achieved this with the love and support of family and friends – and my own inner guidance. When I look back at these experiences, some of which were very difficult, I am grateful for the wisdom and compassion I have gained. This experience has also helped me have a better understanding of what my patients are experiencing.

When John asked me to contribute a naturopathic perspective to the book, I really dug my heels in and I was the busiest I had been in a long time. Thanks to John's original vision and my contributions, we are now presenting a more comprehensive approach to health and fitness than has ever been presented before.

When I look at my life with John, my three wonderful children, loving friends and family, a successful naturopathic practice and now this book which provides a chance for people to experience new levels of health – I cannot express the gratitude I feel.

Life is a continuous adventure that requires mental, emotional, physical and spiritual stamina. I trust that this book will help you accomplish this.

– Karen Jensen, April, 1998

Acknowledgments

To my husband John, the man I always knew was "out there" but wasn't sure I would find; your devotion and support is endless. I would like to thank with all my heart my three wonderful sons for their patience and unspoken acceptance of me during my struggles and the challenges of being a student and during life in general. I would also like to thank my mother and friends who, in the beginning of my studies of naturopathic medicine, thought I was crazy but stood by me anyway; and my ex-husband who, without his undying support and love of the children, made it possible for me to accomplish what I did.

I offer thanks to God, spirit and the universe for the guidance and love that enabled me to survive the painful and tragic death of my then fiancé. His death made me really search inside myself for who and what I wanted to be when I grew up. It was God who gave me the courage to go for my dreams. Finally, I would like to thank my patients and the readers of this book for having the courage and commitment to explore alternative health and for making "optimum health" your goal.

– Karen Jensen

I would like to begin by thanking Deanna Silvester for being there in the early days of the sport. Thanks to Dr. Banister of

Simon Fraser University who introduced me to the merits of training scientifically; thanks to Dr. Lawrence Chan, my first chiropractor and naturopath; and to Detlef Kuhnel and his family who looked after me in 1985 while I raced in Europe during the summer. I would also like to thank the various sponsors who have been so kind as to support me through the years. Thanks to the gang at AVIA Canada, Derrill and Liia Herman of Professional Health Products, Flora and their Floradix Formula, and Jeff Shug of Coggs Frameworks.

I would like to thank the Mahanta for bringing my wife and co-author into my life. Words cannot express the joy and love I feel for her. I wish everyone could find a person such as her to share their life with.

Finally, thanks to *alive* books for embracing this project and being patient while we wrote and tried to meet deadlines. We would especially like to acknowledge the support of Lucy Kenward, Paul Razzell and Catherine Southwood whose support and assistance went beyond the call of duty. Julie Cheng, thank you for tracking down all those permissions. As instrumental as these people were in bringing this book to life, the final product remains our sole responsibility.

To you, the reader, we hope you enjoy this book and find it informative. But remember, put it down from time to time and get out in the fresh air and enjoy being fit and healthy!

– John Winterdyk

Introduction

If you have ever wanted to know just what you are made of and if you ever wanted to feel your body working as a harmonious whole – then this book is for you.

Scan the shelves of any bookstore or newsstand and you will quickly see that health and fitness are popular topics. Scores of publications cover every sports and health-related subject for teens, adults and seniors – from swimming and running to nutrition, training and healing.

Why such a plethora of material? Health and fitness are easily two of the most important concerns people have today. And why not? Maintaining good health and physical fitness directly enhances well-being, improves our immune system, enables us to participate more actively in life and research has shown that it can even prolong life. Staying active and healthy can even reduce the likelihood that you will need medical attention.

In this book we will show you how to attain *optimum health* using an integrated approach to physical fitness, nutrition and a positive mental outlook. If you're a novice, we will demystify the world of cross training and competition and help you to develop a training and nutrition program that suits your personal goals and abilities. If you're a more experienced athlete, we offer detailed advice on how to continually improve your performance and fine-tune the skills you have already. No matter what your level of commitment or ability, you will find practical answers to the following questions:

- How do I monitor my progress so that I train efficiently?
- How do I get the "most" out of the time I have available for training?
- How do I focus my goals and keep motivated throughout the year?
- How much time do I need to train for a triathlon?
- Do I really need to change my eating habits?
- What is a "healthy" nutrition program?
- Do I really need supplements?
- Are there natural substances that will help me perform better?
- As an athlete, what do I need to know about environmental toxins?
- Is there a difference between strength training and endurance training?
- Why should I consider alternative health options?
- Do Chinese herbs, vitamins and homeopathics really work?
- Am I too old to get in shape?

We base our discussion of fitness on the triathlon because, aside from being one of the fastest growing sports in the world, virtually everyone has done one or all of the activities (swim, bike, run) at some time in their life. It is also one of the few sports which requires you to use all your major muscle groups and to exercise aerobically and anaerobically.

Furthermore, multi-disciplinary training offers many advantages that cannot be had when you devote yourself exclusively to a single sport. These advantages include:

1. *Total body fitness and awareness.* If you have ever tried a new activity you'll recall that you discovered muscles you never knew you had! Of course they were there all along, it's just that you seldom call on them to perform in any significant way. Exercise can reveal our strengths and weaknesses. With a little more attention to the way your body feels, you'll acquire a new awareness of just how fit and healthy you are.

   By participating in a multisporting event you'll develop muscular endurance and strength, improve your range of flexibility, strengthen your cardiovascular system (aerobic and anaerobic), probably alter your body fat composition and physical appearance, as well as keep your weight in check. Above all, you will experience a new awareness of who and what you are.

2. *Minimal risk of injury.* Runners often suffer from shin splints, swimmers from shoulder problems, and cyclists from lower back and knee problems. The primary causes of all these sport-specific injuries is overuse of some, and neglect of other muscle groups. Triathletes exercise all the major muscle groups and keep the body in a better state of physical balance, hence, fewer injuries.

3. *Variety.* Have you ever noticed how as the seasons change many people change their activities to complement the season? We like winter for cross-country skiing and summer for hiking. We use these activities to add variety to our regular exercise regime. Being a triathlete allows you to participate in at least three different activities all year-round. In addition, you can vary the intensity, duration and the number of workouts per week or month. The variety also reduces boredom – and the chance that you will abandon your exercise program.

   Since one of the major themes of this book is that you should develop your own program for fitness and health, we will give you guidelines and sample programs with which you can construct your own regimen based on your own interests, aims and abilities. Training should be fun and make you feel great. Ultimately, only you can judge how much and which activities are right for you. We will simply provide you with the essential tools to help you on your way.

In some of the more sport-specific chapters (Chapters 5 through 8) we address the key elements of swimming, cycling, running and strength training. We also tell you all you need to know about preparing for competition. You might feel that participating in a friendly race is not your style or that you do not enjoy the angst of competition. Hopefully, by the time you finish reading this book you will see that you can compete in a way that is in keeping with your temperament.

Just as it it possible to be well-fed but poorly-nourished, it is also possible to become *less* healthy by exercising too much. If you try to incorporate fitness into your lifestyle but start out too ambitiously and incur some injury, you may be discouraged from continuing with the sport. Smart training involves finding a balance between the limits of your body, proper nutrition and emotional well-being. Each of these elements will be discussed in detail later.

Our holistic approach to a healthy and active lifestyle stresses the importance of a properly functioning body. As we all know, your body requires fuel in order to function and you will learn how important it is not only to train your body but how to look after it in a way that promotes health. Nutrition, therefore, is a key element of good health and we will examine it in detail in Chapters 9, 10 and 11.

Karen draws on her extensive clinical knowledge as a naturopath to provide insight into optimum health and nutrition that has never before appeared in a book of this type. The optimum health guidelines offered in the naturopathic portion of the book can be used by everyone, from the elite athlete to the weekend fitness enthusiast.

If you have ever wanted to know just what you were made of; if you have ever wanted to feel your body working as a harmonious whole – then this book is meant for you.

Chapter 1

Motivation and Mental Toughness

WHERE ARE THE STARTING BLOCKS?

What motivates people? What gets them out of the armchair and into those running shoes? The *Oxford Dictionary* defines motivation as "stimulating the interest of a person in an activity." The stimuli often come from friends, family members, teachers, or some individuals whom we hold in high regard – these are all external factors. While these elements may play a role, it is the inner passion that will not only motivate you, but also sustain you.

· Those who believe they can and those who believe they can't are both right.

· When you perform without tension you always do better.

· Direct your energies toward those things that can best help you reach your peak.

· Develop your own goals and your own way of achieving them.

In order to sustain your drive, you need inner motivation. Motivation involves a determination to achieve your goals and to follow your passions, and a commitment to be your best. If you are motivated only by the outcome, you are relying on something you cannot control. And, in spite of all your hard work, you may not attain the external goal and so you may lose your motivation.

Few people, however, ever learn to summon motivation on command. Through self-observation and a positive mental state, you can attain virtually any level of performance you set your mind to. To achieve this state, you need to:

- ► Be responsible for everything. Learn from "failure." Be optimistic.
- ► Set realistic goals and re-evaluate them from time to time.
- ► Use relaxation and visualization exercises to eliminate stress.
- ► Maintain a healthy diet to ensure a sound emotional state.
- ► Remember that only a few things in life are *really* important, so be sure to have fun and see humor in what might otherwise lead to discouragement.
- ► Develop a lifestyle that works for you and make it a ritual.
- ► The driving force in your life should be excellence, quality and satisfaction in knowing you did your best rather than comparing yourself to others or striving only for external success.
- ► Focus on what you can control – the present moment and your attitude.

If you can learn to master these elements then your energy will flow more easily and strongly. When you can perform without tension, you will always do better.

KNOWING YOURSELF AND DEFINING YOUR GOALS

Often the most difficult part of success is determining exactly what you want. It is surprising how many people go through life without setting clearly defined goals for themselves. Therefore, it is important to take some time to understand yourself and discover your passions before you reach for your dreams.

Now try the following exercise to fine-tune your goals. Find a quiet place where you can reflect and write down your responses (they are better put on paper than in a computer because pen and paper are a more personal medium).

STEP 1

Recall an event, or incident, in which you achieved a particular goal or performed exceptionally well. The idea is not to focus on the event but on how it affected you. Then, in the center of the page, jot down the experience. Draw a box, square or circle around it to indicate it was a significant experience. Leave plenty of room around the item so that you can add additional information.

STEP 2

Now sit back and relive the experience. Recall as many details around the event as you can. Was it sunny? What type of setting was it? Were there others around? What were you wearing? Once you are in that place, recall how you felt. What kind of personal experiences accompanied the positive experience? Did you feel joy? Did you feel a sense of relief or a sense of lightness? Did you feel a sense of inner peace or inner power? Jot down a few of your key feelings around the main experience.

TAKING STOCK

Here are some questions for you and the people around you to consider:

1. What level of fitness do I want to have by this time next year?

2. Do I have the necessary commitment to meet my objectives?

3. Am I willing to change my current eating habits and try new activities?

4. Am I likely to measure my achievements by my own yardstick, or will I rate myself against the achievements of others?

5. How will my involvement in holistic fitness impact on my life?

6. What will I sacrifice in order to achieve my goals?

7. How will my involvement affect others (family members, friends, employer and colleagues) in my life? How do their goals and current priorities fit with mine?

8. What are the advantages of training for competition over training for health? Is there some other way I could be involved in a fitness program that might reap more benefits to me and my family?

STEP 3

Once again, focus your mind on those things in your life that are associated with your peak experience. What events contributed to the experience? Arrange these items around the points identified in Step 1. Connect the elements with arrows to show cause and effect.

STEP 4

Now focus directly on the event and recall the things you deliberately did in order to accomplish the task. For example, if your peak race involved an Olympic distance triathlon, what was your training regimen? What kind of equipment did you use? What type of tapering was involved? Did you follow any particular diet? Answering these types of questions is easier when you keep a training log (see Chapter 12).

Repeat this procedure in order to analyze the other great events or achievements in your life. Such events might be work related, family related, or school related. As you reflect on your schematic diagram, you might find some of the points irrelevant and disjointed. This is completely normal.

A commitment to healthy living requires confidence and self-knowledge. Often, though, people's view of themselves is determined by the judgments of others around them and this can all too easily lead to a negative self-image. For many, life represents little more than a series of performances which are judged by others. They begin by needing acceptance from their parents, followed by acceptance from friends, partners, teachers, colleagues and so on. In order to achieve optimum health, then, you must overcome any negative self-image you may have. Fear of failure (anxiety about not being able to meet an objective) and fear of success (anxiety about achieving a goal) are the largest barriers to active living. You can choose to give in to these fears or you can use them to your advantage. You must believe in yourself in order to be truly healthy and achieve your goals.

I learned this lesson the hard way. Physically, I was prepared to finish in the top three at a World Triathlon Championship for several years, but it took four attempts before I finally earned a place on the podium. That was the year I overcame my fear of success. Instead of training only to be physically stronger and faster than my competitors, I began to believe in myself. Even a fall in the early part of the race did not shake my confidence. I knew that I could succeed, and I did.

Fear of failure can usually be limited by taking a proactive role in life and by following these fundamental rules:

1. Seek expert assistance to help you overcome the weaknesses you have in training, racing, work or your relationships.

2. Be patient. When starting any new activity, there are bound to be setbacks. You must keep your sense of humor and always remember the "big picture" – this will keep any setbacks in perspective.

3. Look at your experiences in a positive and motivating way. In other words, *stay optimistic.*

4. Develop your own goals and your own way of achieving them. Do not let anyone else dictate your objectives.

5. Have faith in yourself and in what you are doing. Being somewhat hedonistic and self-focused can be very healthy. Follow your inner voice.

6. Be open to different ways of attaining your goals. Instead of making the Ironman your first goal, go for the 5 km run, then the mini-triathlon, and so on. Have a grand vision but also include smaller goals along the way.

We have personal success when we live and act in accordance with what we believe and value. Sometimes "success" may be stopping to help a friend or needy person (e.g., in the 1986 Ironman Canada Tom Price stopped to help lead runner Dave Kirk when he collapsed). Continually remind yourself of your values and be true to yourself, not to some external abstract.

A final note about fear. Research has shown that our bodies cannot really distinguish between anxiety and excitement: both have similar physiological effects (e.g., increased heart rate, perspiration, butterflies in the stomach and indigestion). If you are experiencing anxiety, therefore, then treat it as *excitement* which will help you to smile and see the humor of the situation. You will also be more likely to enjoy the activity and will look forward to the next one!

What motivates each of us varies from person to person. This is why we do not believe in any set programs. Rather, with some basic tools you can develop your own training and lifestyle program (see Chapter 4). We encourage you to think about some of the ideas shared in this chapter: they represent the fundamentals for "psyching for the sport" and maintaining an active lifestyle. Go out there and enjoy the benefits of feeling great in body, mind, and spirit! As the Alberta Triathlon motto proclaims "Dare to tri." If you don't, you cannot grow and discover all the wonderful potential you have within. We wish you success, sound health and much happiness in your new lifestyle.

Chapter 2

It's About Time

In order to become a "successful" athlete you need to make a time and lifestyle commitment. Triathlons and cross training involve more than one sport and so you need to train perhaps a little more than a single-sport specialist. If you see physical activity as part of your lifestyle, then spending five or more hours a week on fitness should not seem like a lot. What is more, research shows that people also spend a lot of time doing things that may not always be necessary. True enough, sometimes you just need to relax, but how many hours a week do you spend doing the following common activities?

· A few hours a week are all you need to lead a healthy and active lifestyle. The payoff in well-being and vitality will be worth the small investment in time.

▸ watching television

▸ taking coffee breaks

▸ commuting to and from work via car, bus or train

▸ working overtime

Considering the time you spend doing certain non-essential things, you can see how easy it would be to free up at least five or six hours a week which need not detract from your family, work or other necessary commitments. A few hours are all you need to lead a healthy and active lifestyle. The payoff in well-being and vitality will be worth the small investment in time.

One of my favorite examples of a time management expert is a fellow triathlete. He has a full-time job and a very successful business on the side. He is happily married and father of a fine young daughter. Despite all these demands on his time, he trains regularly, participates in triathlons and does very well to boot! Such was not always the case. Before getting into triathlons his weight hovered around 210 pounds and he could not swim the width of a pool, let alone run around the parking lot at the local mall. As he describes it, he woke up one morning to the realization that his emotional and physical health were deteriorating quickly. He decided at that moment to turn his life around. He immediately began exercising, eating well and learning all he could about health and fitness. Today, breakfast and lunch are eaten either on the way to work or while working. Before work he usually fits in a training session, then another at noon, and depending on the time of year another one after work. Yet he still manages to be home for dinner and spend time with his family in the evenings. While his lifestyle may not be ideal for everyone, he is an example of someone who made a conscious decision to alter his life in order to achieve concrete results.

Another good acquaintance regularly runs back and forth to work – a mere dozen miles each way! If this were not enough, he swims several thousand meters before going to work and often squeezes in a bike ride in the evening. This individual holds a number of Canadian long distance running records. In 1996 he finished fourth in his age group (50–54) at the Hawaii Ironman. Yet at one time he was a fairly sedentary person.

These two examples may be considered somewhat eccentric or excessive but the point is that in spite of their busy lives, these people found the time to do the training they felt necessary to achieve their goals. One of the keys to their success has not only been good time management, but an ability to make the most of their time. The key to training then, is not just quantity but quality.

Chapter 3

Fitness Isn't Just for Youngsters

Aging is a process of human development that happens to us all. The physical changes are inevitable: the body burns calories more slowly, maximum heart rate lowers, bodily strength and power decline and recovery from strenuous activity takes longer. So why fight the unavoidable? Why not grow old gracefully? Fortunately for the aging population, an increasing body of evidence indicates we have much more control over how we age than is commonly believed.

· As you age, your muscles naturally lose their suppleness. This can be greatly alleviated if you keep active and use your body in ways that promote flexibility.

· A simple change in diet can improve your capacity to process oxygen which translates to better performance in endurance events.

· By keeping your training interesting and stimulating, you will continue to enjoy it and the likelihood of reaching your short- and long-term goals will improve.

Canadian demographic data reveals that we are an aging population. In 1971 only 8.5 percent of the population was sixty-five years of age or older. In 1986 it rose to 10.7 percent and by the year 2001 it is projected to be 14 percent. In *Boom, Bust and Echo*, David Foot notes that in 1996 the Canadian baby boomers (those born between 1947 and 1966) totaled 9.8 million, or approximately 33 percent of the population. Their needs and expectations are changing and there is a large need to provide specialized services for them.

As we age there will be an increasing need for seniors' caregivers and an expectation to combine longevity with good health. Unfortunately, official health statistics reveal that there were more overweight adults in 1991 than in 1985 and sadly, Canadians are spending more time in hospitals than ever before. With many of the 9.8 million baby boomers now in their fifties, health care is a major issue. Our health care system is in crisis and as all of the boomers will be seniors by 2010, the demands on the health care system will be stretched beyond capacity.

These trends shouldn't frighten us. The simple proactive measures discussed in this chapter will go a long way to helping you maintain a healthy and active lifestyle well into your senior years. Consider these popular myths about growing old.

MYTHS

1. *Nothing can be done about aging.* By returning to settings similar to those you knew when you were in your twenties, thirties, or forties, you can become mentally and physiologically "younger." It is a well-documented fact that older people feel better and more youthful when around younger people. Being involved in an active lifestyle is one means of retarding aging.

2. *If you want to live longer and be healthy you have to give up all your favorite habits.* As we age, our priorities for life, health and happiness also evolve. They are usually dictated by our life experiences.

   You may feel, however, that you have to give up your favorite habits as you get older. Simply because you get slower with age, and your recovery time takes a little longer doesn't mean you have to give up an active, competitive lifestyle. While you may not be able to race as frequently as when you were younger, for example, there is no reason not to be more selective in choosing races.

   I retired from competitive racing several years ago but I still participate in an occasional race. In 1997, I decided to enter a race for fun. I used the opportunity to catch up with old friends, share stories, and yes, to see if I still had what it takes. It was the most relaxed I had ever been before an event, and hanging out with my old friends was most heartwarming. (And yes, I had a great race.) So, you do not have to give up your active lifestyle. In fact, in many ways it can be enriched!

3. *Good health and a long life is possible only if you start working at it when you are young.* A number of years ago my ex-father-in-law, who had been sedentary for most of his life began to "feel his age." His doctor told him that all he needed to do was to be a little more active. Immediately, he joined a fitness club and began to jog. Soon after, he started feeling and acting younger. His attitude became more upbeat, he lost some of his extra weight, and the exercise improved his sense of balance, his body tone and his circulation. Eventually he went on to run his first-ever marathon and placed in his age group (60–64). Everyone who knows him has commented on his "transformation." He has become an inspiration among his friends and continues to lead a healthy, happy and active life. So, no matter how old you are, you are capable of improving your physical and emotional well-being.

MYTHS AND BARRIERS ARE MEANT TO BE BROKEN!

► In 1985, Portugal's Carlos Lopes set the marathon record in 2:07:12. He was thirty-eight. At the 1984 Los Angeles Olympic marathon, Lopes beat thirty-seven men who were at least ten years younger than himself.

► In 1981, American swimmer Lance Larson (forty-one) beat all his previous fourteen world records – the last of which he won in 1961!

► In 1988, Susan Fraenkel of South Africa became the oldest woman to swim the English Channel. She was nearly forty-seven. The oldest man to do so was Clifford Batt of Australia who was nearly sixty-eight when he swam across in 1989.

- And then there is Bernie Hogan of Australia. In 1976 he set a world record for the 100-meter dash. He has also won the World Championship in the 100-meter and 200-meter dash in 1977, 1979, 1981, 1983, 1991 and 1993. In 1993 he was seventy-three years of age! He still trains five to six days per week. And how does he keep motivated? "Sports," says Bernie, "has become a way of life."

- Roman Jezek, of Canada, won the 80+ age category at the 1996 ITU Amateur Triathlon World Championship. His race time would also have been good enough to win him the 75–79 age category!

- Scott Tinley, at age thirty-five, won the Ironman Canada in 1992. In the process he beat three-time winner Ray Browning and over 1,000 other hopefuls. Tinley's time – 8:27! Do you need more convincing? It took until 1996 before two "young bucks" were finally able to break his course record!

- Forty-year-old Dave Scott, the six-time Hawaii Ironman winner, returned to the lava fields of Hawaii in 1994 after a five-year hiatus and finished a strong second to a much younger Greg Welch.

- At the World Masters' Games in 1994, in Brisbane, a woman nearly ninety years of age competed in a swimming event!

The list could go on but the point is clear. While aging is a natural process, there are many things we can do to maximize our enjoyment.

THE TORTOISE AND THE HARE

A 1995 Canadian study compared the results of strength training in elderly and younger athletes. The study revealed some noteworthy findings. While the younger group experienced improved muscle growth during the first few weeks of training, the masters (older) group did not start to blossom until halfway into the eight-week program. The elders improved their strength by an amazing sixty-one percent! So, while you may not get results overnight, patience and dedication to an active lifestyle will pay off.

CONTROLLING THE AGING PROCESS

Some of the tell-tale signs of aging are reduced flexibility, decline in strength and loss of cardiovascular efficiency. While these symptoms begin at different ages, it is usually in our mid-thirties that our bodies begin to show diminishing returns. Thanks to science and a growing body of knowledge about human physiology, however, if you are thirty-five you do not have to buy that rocking chair just yet! In fact, by modifying their lifestyle some individuals have actually been able to improve with age.

The key to managing the aging process is to anticipate its causes and to control them using the following techniques: flexibility, endurance through strength training, nutrition, psychology and smart training.

FLEXIBILITY

The literature on stretching is controversial. Stretching guru Bob Anderson has said that we need to stretch regularly to counteract the tightness and inflexibility we experience as a natural part of aging and the cumulative rigors of staying active. Philip Maffetone, one of the "new age" fitness kings, claims there is "no scientific evidence that stretching is helpful." In fact, he argues that aerobic exercise provides the full range of motion needed. The best advice may be to look at nature as a guide. Cats, for example, seldom get injured through regular activity. This is due in part to the fact that cats are excellent stretchers. Our two cats stretch every morning before feeding and stretch regularly throughout the day. Unlike dogs, I have never heard of a cat suffering from joint problems. While there is some risk in generalization, controlled stretching after a light warm-up will help fight stiffness and reduce your chances of injury. Popular stretching activities are t'ai chi, yoga and qi gong. These techniques enhance your flexibility and make you more aware of your body – all by breathing and moving properly.

As we age our muscles naturally lose their suppleness. This can be greatly alleviated if we keep active and use our bodies in ways that promote flexibility.

ENDURANCE THROUGH STRENGTH TRAINING

Since we devote a whole chapter to strength training (see Chapter 8), we will focus our comments here on "maturing" athletes. Unused muscle loses strength and tone with time. Strength training can counteract this process and even improve performance; it will also help you look younger and feel better.

Masters coach Greg Reddan from Australia notes that the benefits of maintaining muscle tone and strength far outweigh any disadvantages. Upper- and lower-body strength significantly affect endurance. Dave Scott, the six-time Ironman winner, is a strong advocate of strength training. He feels it is particularly important for running and endurance activities.

We advocate variety in your program. Use the off-season to focus on strength building. This should be done four days per week with split routines. Pre-season training can be reduced to three days while the race season should involve a general reduction in the number of sets, repetitions and frequency workouts. Table 3.1 gives a suggested program. As always, you should experiment in consultation with your health care practitioner to determine what works best for you.

Table 3.1 ENDURANCE/STRENGTH TRAINING CYCLE
FOR OLDER ATHLETES

OFF-SEASON *(approximately 7 weeks – 4 days/week)*

	MONDAY/THURSDAY	TUESDAY/FRIDAY
WEEKS 1–2	*Lower Body*	*Upper Body*
3 sets × 10 reps	· abdominals	· bent knee sit-ups
	· leg press/squats	· bench press
WEEKS 3–4	· step-ups/lunges	· inclined bench
3 sets × 8 reps	· leg extensions/curls	· shoulder – front/lateral/rear
	· gluts-ham/hip extensions	· bicep curls
WEEKS 5–7	· calf raises	· triceps
3 sets × 6 reps	· lat pulls	· wrist curls

PRE-SEASON *(approximately 6 weeks – 3 days/week)*

	MONDAY	TUESDAY	THURSDAY (CIRCUIT)
WEEKS 1–3	*Lower Body*	*Upper Body*	*Upper/Lower Body*
3 sets × 8 reps	· crunches	· bent knee sit-ups	· leg press/squat
	· step-ups/lunges	· bench press	· bench press
WEEK 4	· leg press/squats	· inclined bench	· step-ups/lunges
3 sets × 10 reps	· leg ext/curls	· shoulder circuit	· inclined bench
	· gluts-ham	· biceps/triceps	· bent arm pull-over
WEEK 5	· calf-raise	· wrist curls	· lateral raise
3 sets × 12 reps			· leg extension
			· leg curls
WEEK 6			· hip flexor
3 sets × 13 reps			· biceps
			· calf raises
			· wrist curls

RACE SEASON *(approximately 4 weeks – 2 days/week)*

	MONDAY	THURSDAY
WEEKS 1-2	*Upper/Lower Body*	*Upper/Lower Body*
3 sets × 15 reps	· leg press/squats	· bench press
	· bench press	· inclined bench
WEEKS 3-4	· leg extensions/curls	· leg extensions/curls
2 sets × 20 reps	· bent arm pull-over	· lats – front/back
	· hip flexor	· triceps
	· biceps	· wrist curls
	· calf raises	

You should also keep the following points in mind:

- Do a proper cool down after every workout.
- If you are feeling a little sore, "chill out" – take it easy.
- Get a regular sports massage to help keep you supple and rejuvenated.
- After a hard workout, do a light workout the next day and then rest the day after that. This will enable you to recover more effectively than taking the day off following a hard workout.

If you have access to the Internet, you'll find comprehensive information for strength training and bodybuilding for master athletes at *http://ageless.athletes.com*. This site is the home of the bimonthly newsletter publication, *MasterTrainer*.

NUTRITION

Since we are what we eat, it should be easy to figure out what is good or bad for us. However, in this hectic world of processed and irradiated foods, mutated hybrids and mass advertisement, things are not so simple anymore. For example, since 1943 the recommended daily allowance (RDA) for protein has been revised at least ten times! Yet the RDAs do not distinguish between dietary requirements for the various adults over the age of 50. It assumes the dietary needs of a 70 year old are the same as those of a 55 or 90 year old. Most experts agree, however, that dietary needs of people in their fifties are different from people in their seventies. Here, we offer some basic guidelines to help you meet your nutritional requirements.

Many older books recommend a dietary program consisting of fifteen percent protein, thirty percent (or less) fats, and sixty to seventy percent carbohydrates. The rationale for a high-carbohydrate diet was that since our bodies use stored carbohydrates (glycogen) for energy, it makes sense to carbo-load. Dr. Barry

Sears and Dr. Philip Maffetone, however, argue something quite different. They suggest your dietary balance should be forty percent carbohydrates, thirty percent protein, and thirty percent fat. The technical reasons for this ratio are beyond the scope of this book. Suffice it to say that this change was partly inspired by the research which garnered the 1982 Nobel Prize for Medicine.

The food we eat affects our eicosanoids, powerful hormones which control the rate of oxygen transfer to muscle cells. As Sears describes it in *Enter the Zone,* you can produce either "good" or "bad" eicosanoids by virtue of what you eat. By switching to the 40:30:30 formula you can improve your capacity to process oxygen which translates to better performance in endurance events and reduces your risk of lactic acid build-up. For example, Sam Graci, author of *The Power of Superfoods,* suggests you might want to experiment with a diet of fifty-five percent carbohydrates, twenty-five percent low-fat proteins, and twenty percent fats. He recommends combining this diet with a drink composed of several organic, nutrient-rich land- and sea vegetables for maximum detoxification, blood cleansing and bowel regulation.

Regardless of your age, you should consider a number of factors when determining your caloric intake. These include gender, body size, metabolic rate, underlying medical conditions and food preferences. Some of the essential issues surrounding this topic are covered in Chapter 9. Here we offer a number of fundamental nutrition guidelines that any masters athlete (over 35 years of age) can and should consider.

There are, of course, other dietary practices recommended for active people.

► Enjoy a variety of foods that are natural, minimally processed (if at all), and preferably organic. Not only will you obtain more nutritional value from what you eat but you are less likely to take in unnecessary salt and other additives often found in processed foods.

- ► Be sure to keep fats, proteins and wholesome carbohydrates in the recommended proportions. Refer to Chapter 9.

- ► Maintain a healthy body weight. Obesity is not a normal condition of aging.

- ► Drink more pure water (e.g., distilled, bottled or reverse osmosis). It is almost impossible to drink too much. Thirst is a poor indicator of your fluid needs so you should drink a comfortable amount at regular intervals whether you are thirsty or not.

- ► Consume caffeine in the form of coffee or tea in moderation. Given the popularity of coffee these days you might be interested in reading Peter D'Adamo's book, *Eat Right 4 Your Type*. If your blood is type A, coffee is highly beneficial but not black tea. On the other hand, if your blood is type O, you should avoid coffee and black tea.

- ► Consume alcohol only in moderation.

- ► Do not smoke.

- ► Limit simple sugars like table sugar and sweets.

- ► Include vitamin D in your diet; it is essential for proper calcium absorption. As we age, we lose our natural ability to synthesize vitamin D from the sun.

- ► Ensure that you obtain vitamin B6; it helps to support the nervous and immune systems. Vitamin E also has a positive effect on the immune system.

- ► Take vitamin C. According to some research, vitamin C has been shown to protect the elderly against the potential damage of ultraviolet light and has been associated with a reduced risk of cataracts.

On a final note, recent research has found that as we age we can minimize recovery time from strenuous exercise by consuming quick-energy foods shortly after the activity. Quick-energy foods should include complex carbohydrates such as bagels, pasta and potatoes. These will not send your blood sugar levels through the roof. Small amounts of protein and fat are also advisable if you have been working out for more than two hours. Simple sugars like soda pop and candy bars will only give you temporary relief and will not aid in a speedy recovery.

PSYCHOLOGY

Age is simply a state of mind! Who has not heard this expression before? As you age the mind-body link plays an increasingly important role in who you are, what you are, and how you feel. The concept of "old" and "young" is in many respects a false duality. While you may no longer keep up with the youngsters, if you learn to focus on the present, rather than on what was or what might be, you can continue to feel just as young and gain just as much satisfaction from being a part of an event as anyone else. Learn to develop short-term goals (e.g., daily and weekly training) to help you stay "in the moment." Your long-term goals can simply be the races you wish to participate in. In addition, use visualization and relaxation techniques to help you cope with reality and aging. We will discuss visualization and relaxation in Chapter 13.

TRAINING

Developing your own program based on flexibility, endurance, strength, nutrition and psychology will improve your health and fitness for many years to come. No matter what your age, your body and mind will respond to a well designed training program.

Deepak Chopra's *Ageless Body, Timeless Mind* provides a number of keys to help you to actively master your training.

► Be sure to listen to your body's wisdom. Heed signs of fatigue such as muscle soreness, loss of sleep, feeling unusually agitated, and other warning signals.

- Live in the present. Focus all of your being into everything you think and do. When you do, time becomes timeless. Sometimes in a race when I was totally absorbed in what I was doing, I lost all sense of time and effort. For most of us, reaching this state takes practice but once you have experienced it, you will want to experience it again. While it is good to have long-term goals, focusing on what you can do today is not only fulfilling but it can help you attain your long-term goals.

- Take time to be silent. Pay attention to your inner life.

- Enjoy what you are doing. If you do not enjoy swimming or running, why do it? By keeping your training interesting and stimulating, you will continue to enjoy it and the likelihood of reaching your short- and long-term goals will improve.

Given that as we age our bodies tend to become more sensitive to impurities, anyone serious about their well-being might want to look carefully at the growing body of research into organic foods and nutrition. An excellent, very readable book is *The New Nutrition* by Michael Colgan. Now we are ready to move on and develop a personalized training program. Grab your gear and let's go!

Chapter 4

Developing A Personalized Training Program

Do you ever find it frustrating following a generic workout – the type often found in sports magazines? If so, it is probably because the program does not account for your particular needs, health and level of expertise. Developing a training program which suits all of your needs and abilities is easier than you might think. While there is nothing wrong with getting a personal coach, for example, the self-discovery and satisfaction that come from developing your own program will be more than worth the effort. By following the basic principles listed below, you can tailor a training regimen to fit your goals, your level of conditioning and health. The end result may look somewhat similar to the sample programs provided, but it will be tailored to you.

The first step in developing a personalized training program is to ask yourself the following questions about your present abilities, aims and interests:

► What is the current state of my health? If it has been more than a year since your last

· A smart training program is divided into segments that allow you to make progressive improvements.

· The self-discovery and satisfaction that come from developing your own program will reward you far more than if you merely followed a generic workout.

· Cross training involves you in a variety of activities so you avoid the risk of boredom and the subsequent abandonment of your exercise program.

· Research has shown that aerobic activity is beneficial to the nervous and circulatory systems, and it improves hormonal balance and the metabolism of fatty acids.

physical, you should get a check-up before you do any training. Let your doctor know what you are planning to do and get a full physical examination. Do not proceed any further until you have a clean bill of health.

- ▸ What kind of injuries have I had? For example, after trying to run twenty to thirty kilometers a week do you begin to develop knee pains, or does your shoulder act up when you swim a great distance? Do you have a recurring injury or ache that flares up when you overdo it? If so, part of the problem may have to do with the proportion of aerobic versus anaerobic activity in your training.

- ▸ What kind of time do I *really* have for maintaining a healthy lifestyle?

- ▸ What are my current skill levels in the activities I want to pursue?

- ▸ What would I like to get out of my program? For example, do I want to lose weight, tone my body, or compete in certain races?

- ▸ How sound is my athletic background? Check your level of fitness against the standards found in the Appendix to determine your physical strengths and weaknesses.

- ▸ How competitive have I been in the past? Are my significant others aware of my forthcoming lifestyle change? How supportive are they?

A smart training program is divided into segments that allow you to make progressive improvements. You will have different objectives for different weeks and seasons and for this reason it is wise to break your training into cycles. Depending on your objectives, you may want to plan short month-long cycles or longer four-year "quadrennia" like the Eastern European Olympians. Since doing the same type of workout day after day will only enable you to reach a certain level, cyclical training (see Figure 4.2) will enable you to improve and at the same time reduce the risk of boredom and injury.

STRETCHING

Stretching should be part of any smart training program. With your muscles relaxed and the blood flowing easily through your body, you will be less likely to injure yourself and you will reach your optimum health much sooner. There are stretching exercises designed for overall flexibility as well as stretches that are specific to each sport. Bear in mind that you can easily hurt yourself if you do not stretch properly, so read the following guidelines carefully before incorporating stretching into your training program.

▸ Stretching should always follow your warm-up. Your body's core temperature should be elevated before engaging in a static stretch.

▸ Stretching should be done with a focused mind. Concentrate on what you are doing so that you can feel your body's response and you don't overdo it.

▸ Stretching should be accompanied by proper breathing. As you stretch, breathe into it and feel your muscle relax. Anyone who has practiced yoga or t'ai chi, will be familiar with this principle.

▸ Move into a stretch slowly and hold it at the point of comfortable tension. As you hold the stretch (fifteen or more seconds) you can breathe into it then slowly release the tension. The stretch should never feel uncomfortable.

▸ After you have completed any exercise, take a few minutes to stretch the muscles you have just used. For example, after a run stretch your calves, hamstrings, quadriceps and lower back.

EXERCISE AND MUSCLE TYPES — AEROBIC AND ANAEROBIC

When developing a training program you should be aware of the distinction between aerobic and anaerobic workouts. In recent years the fitness catchphrase has been "quality not quantity." Unfortunately, many people have taken this to mean that training harder is better. Such is not always the case. Too much intense exercise can lead to anaerobic excess, which is discussed below.

The relative proportion of aerobic to anaerobic muscle varies from person to person depending on their physical make-up and the type of activities they pursue. Athletes in certain sports, such as long-distance running, show a larger ratio of aerobic to anaerobic muscle fibers than, say, football players. Endurance athletes have more slow-twitch muscle fibers in their legs, shoulders and arms (the muscle groups being specifically trained for endurance) than sprinters or power lifters who focus their development on their fast-twitch muscle fibers.

Your fast-twitch muscle fibers are divided into two types, each of which is used during a different phase of athletic activity. The first group of fast-twitch muscles uses the body's naturally produced creatine phosphate to propel the body anaerobically over short distances in a short amount of time (think of sprinters running the 100 meter dash in ten seconds or less). When this "firecracker" has been depleted and the first group of fast-twitch muscles fatigues, the body's second group of fast-twitch muscles kicks in. By burning the glycogen in circulation in the body, this second group of muscles moves from an anaerobic state to an aerobic one (think of middle-distance runners covering 1,500 meters in a couple of minutes). Fast-twitch muscle fibers, then, produce energy mostly anaerobically but fatigue over the short-to-moderate term. The enduring slow-twitch muscle fibers contract slowly when breaking down the body's fat-stored glycogen to produce energy aerobically. By definition, slow-twitch muscle fibers fatigue more slowly than fast-twitch fibers. Marathon runners, for example, rely on their slow-twitch fibers to sustain them over the long haul.

What is not clear is whether training produces changes to muscle composition or maximizes a genetic predisposition. Research has shown that significant aerobic training can improve the oxidative capacity of fast-twitch muscle fibers. Yet training does not seem to have the same effect on extending the anaerobic capacity of fast-twitch muscle fibers, which can only supply all-out energy for about two minutes. Aerobic exercise conditions your heart and circulatory system – anaerobic exercise does not. For this reason, training programs now focus on building strength and endurance by exercising sport-specific muscle groups. Your training and your diet will depend on the ratio of your aerobic to anaerobic muscles because each muscle type has different energy, mineral and electrolyte sources (see Table 4.1).

Table 4.1 MUSCLE TYPE CHARACTERISTICS

	AEROBIC	ANAEROBIC
Dominant source of energy	fatty acids	glucose
Muscle reaction	slow	fast
Function	endurance	speed
Metabolism facilitator	iron	pantothenic acid
Electrolyte source	sodium	potassium

Since the body is comprised primarily of aerobic muscle, a balanced health and fitness program requires that *seventy-five to eighty-five percent of exercise and activity be aerobic, that is, working out at sixty to seventy-five percent of your maximum heart rate* (your anaerobic threshold). As some experts have described it, aerobic activity should feel like "guilt-producing fun." Aerobic activities tend to be done over extended time and at a steady pace. Therefore, rowing, swimming, cycling, running, rollerblading and cross-country skiing are activities well suited to the development of aerobic muscles – assuming you are not racing.

Anaerobic activity, aside from racing, involves working the muscles "without air" in all-out efforts and usually for a short time. Examples include an intense weight lifting effort or a sprint, whether it's running, cycling or swimming. Anaerobic activity should occupy fifteen to twenty percent of your training time.

Research has clearly shown that aerobic activity is beneficial to the nervous system and circulatory system, it improves hormonal balance and enhances the metabolism of fatty acids. When your aerobic system is working well and you are following a healthy nutrition program, your blood sugar level will be stable and your brain will function normally. An imbalance of blood sugar usually results in mood swings, fatigue and weight fluctuations.

Although our anaerobic system represents a smaller proportion of our muscle fibers, it must also be exercised in order for a person to be fit and healthy. For elite or competitive athletes this is seldom a problem. What is a problem is the amount of time some athletes spend in an anaerobic state . . . the "no pain, no gain" or "go for the burn" mentality. Just as you can have aerobic excess or deficiency, you can also have too little or too much anaerobic exercise.

Anaerobic deficiency usually manifests itself in an imbalance of the body's chemistry. The symptoms are similar to those of aerobic excess: there is a plateau in progress, you get neither stronger nor faster, and if you are trying to lose weight it is likely you will be unable to shed an ounce – perhaps you will even gain a bit.

Classic symptoms of *anaerobic excess* include: burn-out, proneness to injury, seeing no value in warming up or cooling down, failure to improve performance, craving for sweets and even difficulty waking in the morning. For example, if you ever feel stiff when getting up in the morning it may be because you have been doing more than twenty percent anaerobic activity over a prolonged period of time. By better understanding the relationship between proper aerobic and anaerobic activity, you can better organize, and monitor your training program to suit your needs.

THE BASIC ELEMENTS OF ANY TRAINING CYCLE

A training cycle should offer a variety of activity and enough flexibility to enable you to make progressive improvements in your performance. Training cycles usually build toward a competition or major event, but if you prefer not to race, you can still use the cycle to develop your abilities to their utmost level. The basic elements of any training cycle include:

1. *Building an aerobic base.* Regardless of the sport, you will need to learn the basic techniques and determine the limits of your body. In this first phase you should focus on staying aerobic. Therefore your heart rate should stay approximately ten beats below your maximum aerobic rate during this period. *Duration:* Weeks 1–10 for a sixteen-week program, or eight to nine months for a year-long program (approximately eighty percent of your training cycle).

2. *Anaerobic speed work.* Once you have built a solid fitness and endurance foundation you will be ready to fine-tune your performance – by adding speed and duration to your workouts. Given the demands that anaerobic activity places on your body, this is a relatively short phase. *Duration:* Weeks 11–14 for a sixteen-week program, or approximately six weeks for a year-long program (ten to fifteen percent of your training cycle).

3. *Tapering.* Just before the "big" race athletes will sometimes fall into the trap of pushing themselves to be faster and stronger. This is an example of overtraining and by doing so you run the risk of going into the race without adequate rest. Tapering involves reducing your training load so that your energy levels can be restored in time for the race. *Duration:* One week for a sixteen-week program, or three weeks for a year-long program (five to ten percent of your training cycle).

4. *Peaking and racing!* After you have worked hard and know that you have properly prepared yourself for the challenge, you can enter the event confident you will do well.

5. *Restoration.* After the racing season is over it is time to give your body a rest although we recommend that you engage in *active rest.* Keep active but do things for fun and with low intensity. This

phase can last from a few days to a few weeks depending on the type of program you have developed.

The restoration phase is the area of training most often neglected by athletes. Although we are referring to recovery at the end of a thorough training cycle, the recovery process should also be incorporated into your regular workouts, that is, before and after a workout or race.

Short- and long-term recovery can include a range of passive activities such as hot showers or baths, saunas, short spins, massage, relaxation and stretching, muscle stimulation, ultrasound, sports psychology, t'ai chi, yoga, vitamin and mineral build-up, and the use of adaptogens (see Chapter 14).

Table 4.2 shows a sample year-long training cycle for a triathlete. This cycle begins in December and ends in January, but you can adapt the program to suit your needs and the seasons. Note that it includes all the relevant building blocks: building an aerobic base, anaerobic speedwork, tapering, racing/peaking, and restoration. You might want to think of this as keeping in tune with the cycles of nature in which everything has its proper season. As long as you follow the basic objectives of each stage and monitor your progress against your goals, then you will be able to train with good results.

Remember though, even as the best home requires periodic maintenance, so too will your fitness program. Re-evaluate and fine-tune your program each year to account for age, new interests and life's never-ending challenges.

Table 4.2 TRAINING CYCLE FOR ONE YEAR

Building an Aerobic Base: During this phase you want to build a solid foundation of skills and cardiovascular strength. Therefore, most workouts should be aerobic. Don't get too intense. You will need the drive later in the year.

	ACTIVITY	#/WK	DUR (min)	DIST	FORMAT	OBJECTIVE
DEC	Swim	1	60	2,400 m	Steady	Technique
	Run	2	90	16 km	Steady	Form/technique
	(X-Country Ski)	5–6	60	3×2 km	3 km easy	Form/technique
	Strength Train	2	40–50			Strength lifting
	Aerobics*	1	120			Fun
	Total:	**5–6**	**6:10–6:30 hrs**			
JAN	Swim	1–2	80–100	3–3.5 km	5×200 m	Form/technique
	Run	2	90–135	20–25	Steady	
	(X-Country Ski)		70	14 km	3×3 km	
	Strength Train	2–3	40–60			Power/strength
	Aerobics	1	120			Fun
	Total:	**6–8**	**6:30–8 hrs**			

Anaerobic Speed Work: Now you should start incorporating anaerobic activities into your workout. The balance should be eighty percent aerobic and twenty percent anaerobic. Each workout has a specific purpose.

	ACTIVITY	#/WK	DUR (min)	DIST	FORMAT	OBJECTIVE
FEB	Swim	1	80–100	3–3.5 km	4×200/7×100	
	Swim	1		1,500 m		
	Run	2	100–140	20–28 km	Steady	
	(X-Country Ski)					Form/technique
	Strength Train	3	40–60			Power/stretching
	Aerobics	1	120			Fun
	Total:	**8**	**5:30–7 hrs**			
MAR	Swim	2	80–100	3–3.5 km	More interval	
	Cycle	1	90	45 km	Speed play	
	Cycle	1	70	30 km	Races	
	Run	1	50	12 km	Speed play	
	Run	1	120	25 km	Steady	
	Strength Train	2–3	40–60			Endurance/flexibility
	Aerobics	1	120			Still time for fun!
	Total:	**9–10**	**9:30–10 hrs**			

* skiing, volleyball, speed skating, etc.

Months Five to Six: Follow the same basic regimen as for month four but begin to introduce more speed work as you approach month seven. Speed work involves reducing the total number and duration of workouts and introducing anaerobic workouts. Time, distance and objectives of all activities remain the same. You are simply building your aerobic base, becoming more intense, and working toward peaking.

Racing/Peaking: You have done all the hard work, now you want to stay sharp for the races. Pick your key races and prepare for them. During this phase, training will be a matter of fine-tuning your skills.

	ACTIVITY	#/WK	DUR (min)	DIST	FORMAT	OBJECTIVE
JUN	Swim	2–3	75–120	2.5–7 km	Distance & intervals	Open water swimming
	Cycle	1	150	60–70 km	Some tempo	
	Cycle	2	2 × 60/75	40–50 km	Repeats & hill work	
	Run	3	75–90	15–20 km		Endurance
	Run	3	45–55	10–12 km	3 × 2 km	Sprints
	Aerobics & Strength Training	1	40–60		Light weights & aerobics	
	Total:	**9–10**	**10–12 hrs**			
JUL/	Swim	2	60–90	2.8–3.5 km	Work on drills	
AUG/	Cycle	3	75–150	40–70 km	Work on drills & recovery	
SEP	Run	2	45–80	10–15+ km	Recovery, drills, short intervals	
	Strength/Stretch	1–2	30		Lt. weights	Toning/maintenance
	Total:	**8–9**	**3:30–6 hrs**			

Rest/Restoration: Unless you are doing the Hawaii Ironman or moving to the southern hemisphere, the race season for most northern bound triathletes is over. This is the time to engage in active rest and have fun.

	ACTIVITY	#/WK	DUR (min)	DIST	FORMAT	OBJECTIVE
OCT/ NOV	Swim	1	60	2.5 km	Split your time between staying loose and playing!	
	Cycle	2	40–75	30–45 km		
	Get out the mountain bike or go out and enjoy the changing of the season – play!					
	Run	2	40–75	8–15 km		
	Go out and relax, breathe the crisp air and enjoy nature!					
	X-Training					
	Hiking, roller-blading, walking, squash . . . discover the joy of staying fit and having fun!					
Total:		**5+**	**6 hrs**			

Please note that this chart is based on a year-long commitment to cross training. This chart is intended for athletes who wish to bring themselves to a level where they could participate in Olympic or half-Ironman distance triathlon races. It is also designed to provide variety in your program. Bear in mind that this program is not cast in stone; feel free to modify it to suit your aims and abilities.

STAYING ON TOP OF YOUR GAME ALL YEAR?

Much has been written about staying in peak form throughout the year. While this may be possible, the chances that you would maintain such a lifestyle for very long are rather remote. Just as the moon and the seasons pass through different phases, virtually every natural phenomenon has its own cycles – and so should your training.

Chapter 5

Swimming

In ancient times swimming was practiced for both utilitarian and health reasons. The Greek historian Herodotus (485–425 BC) wrote about the benefits of swimming and in 1603 Japan issued an imperial edict making swimming part of the school curriculum. As one author noted in the publication *Sports in the USSR*, "in swimming, possibly more than in any other sport, a person remembers that he is a child of nature."

· The art of swimming well is to have good stroke efficiency and speed.

· If you have not done much stretching, it will take two to four weeks of at least four sessions weekly before you begin to feel the benefits.

As a vehicle for health and fitness, swimming ranks very highly, although it is probably the most difficult of the three triathlon sports to master. The weaker your technique, the more drag you are likely to create. And drag is your worst enemy when swimming, especially when you realize that water is 1,000 times more dense than air! But what does drag really mean?

If you are six feet tall, weigh 165 pounds and swim 5,280 feet (one mile), you have to pull your body the equivalent of 880 body lengths. Your weight combined with the drag created would have you pulling 132,000 pounds or 66 tons through the water in order to complete the distance. Fortunately, the better your technique, the less drag you will have and the easier it will be to move your body through the water.

It is not possible in this type of book to give all the advice needed to help you become a great swimmer but we will offer some tips which you might consider incorporating into your program. You will need to practice and have someone watch and (ideally) videotape your efforts. The impact of visual feedback can be profound. Until I saw on video how badly I fishtailed, I was unable to correct the problem. Video sessions can also be great for adding a little humor to what you are doing. Perhaps it will put things into perspective – you might even admire how much you have improved.

Four major strokes are used in competitive swimming: the crawl, backstroke, breaststroke and the butterfly. Any of these strokes will suffice in a triathlon but the crawl is the fastest and this is why all competitive triathletes use it. For more information on strokes see Maglischo's excellent book, *Swimming Even Faster* or the 90-minute video *Swimming Skills*. This video offers stroke demonstrations and basic water safety tips. As your technique improves, you will become more efficient, save energy and feel better.

FLEXIBILITY FOR SMOOTHER STROKES

Before you jump into the pool, you should always warm up with some stretching in order to optimize your flexibility. Mitchell Feingold, former consultant to the US cycling team, noted that good physical performance in any sport is based on strength, endurance, speed, coordination and flexibility. Flexibility is the ability of a joint to move through its full range of motion. Poor flexibility is usually due to muscle tightness – a common cause of stress-related injuries.

If you have not done much stretching it will take between two to four weeks of at least four sessions weekly to begin to feel the benefits. Flexibility routines done within two hours of completing a workout or race are helpful. However, do not stretch until after your body has cooled down. Otherwise, you risk over-stretching an already taxed muscle.

According to Maglischo, author of *Swimming Faster* and his sequel, *Swimming Even Faster*, little is actually known about increasing the range of motion in joints. In recent years, there has been a

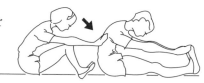

1. *Stretch comfortably as far as you can. The stretcher assistant pushes on the back in the direction of the stretch to extend the limit.*

growing consensus that ballistic stretching (i.e., quick swinging and bending with little time spent holding a position) will not increase your range of motion, whereas static and propriocep-tive neuromuscular facilitation (PNF) will. This stretching technique has been used successfully for years by dancers, gymnasts, track and field athletes, as well as physical and massage therapists.

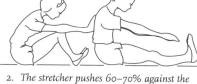

2. *The stretcher pushes 60–70% against the force of the assistant for 6 seconds.*

PNF is a combination of static stretches and isometric contrac-tions. Static stretches slowly force a joint beyond its normal range of motion (e.g., trying to touch your toes) and are held for ten to fifteen seconds. Isometric contractions involve varying the force of muscular contraction and holding the stretch for a short period of time. Ideally these exercises involve a partner who pushes against you to do the isometric part of the PNF movement. Once you reach the limit of your static stretch your partner gently stretches you beyond your normal limit (1). You then apply approximately sixty to sev-enty percent force against your part-ner for six seconds (2). Release the

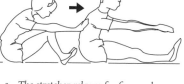

3. *The stretcher relaxes for 6 seconds. The assistant still pushes in the direction of the stretch but not beyond the limit of the stretch.*

4. *Repeat steps 2 and 3 twice more, finishing with the stretch.*

pressure for six seconds (3), then repeat twice more (4). Each exercise should be repeated three to five times, always finishing with the stretch. Our muscles have a natural protection against overstretching. It is known as the stretch reflex. If you attempt to stretch too far or too quickly your muscles will automatically contract to prevent tearing. PNF is an excellent technique to carefully override the stretch reflex. Nevertheless, you should never feel pain.

While the PNF movement can help to significantly increase your range of motion and flexibility, combining static and PNF movements is even better. Many of the top athletes now incorporate flexibility routines into their workouts in order to keep them relatively injury-free, competitive and healthy for a longer time.

CRAWL TECHNIQUE

According to Dr. Ernest Maglischo, there are five key elements to the crawl: the kick, the arm stroke, the timing of the arms and legs, the body position and the breathing.

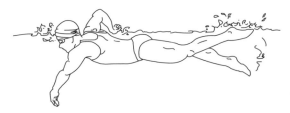

While the flutter kick provides minimal propulsion, when done properly it elevates your torso for a more streamlined body which allows you to maximize the effort you are putting into your stroke. Some coaches recommend using a special flipper aid, which forces you to kick harder and work ankle flexion. Smaller flippers enable a regular swim kick beat. The general rule of thumb is that you should not use swim aids for more than thirty percent of your swim workout. Hand paddles put additional stress on your shoulders while flippers add strain to your lower back and quads.

Hand entry should be about one foot (30 cm) in front of the shoulder, with your palm turned out slightly so that the inside of your middle finger goes into the water first.

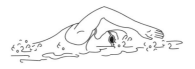

Visualize slipping your hand into the water in front of your shoulder while creating the least amount of drag. This type of entry helps to create lift and allows you to ride higher in the water. The flatter your entry the greater the splash and the slower you go. Also watch that you do not overreach or cross over the imaginary midline that runs from the center vertical axis of your body. Doing so will pull your body out of its streamlined position and will result in the famous fishtail and scissor kicks which only create more drag.

After you slip your entry (or right) arm into the water you want to extend it forward under the water – this is called the *stretch* or *glide.*

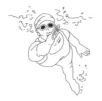

Because your left arm is part way through the propulsion phase, it would not be efficient to begin propelling yourself forward with the entry arm. You want the stretch to be smooth and effortless. The glide should be timed so that as your propelling (left) arm is about to exit, your entry arm is reaching its maximum extension. As you practice this stroke you will naturally develop the body roll you so often hear about. Begin the catch

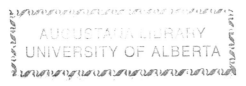

when the entry arm is at its fullest extension.

The *catch* begins just as the left arm has completed its propulsion.

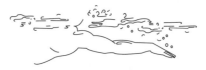

The catch involves flexing your right wrist downward and slightly outward so as to create the lift force. It also helps you to flex the elbow and prepare for the downsweep and pull.

When properly done, the *downsweep* produces a smooth S movement. As your right arm goes down and your elbow remains flexed you get a natural body roll and the right hand will almost automatically slide outward. Only after you have reached your full downward sweep do you begin the insweep or the pull.

The *pull* is the power stroke.

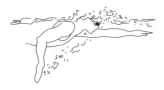

After the downsweep, your right arm should increase in speed. Flex your right hand at the wrist so that you are pulling the water straight back. The pull should begin when your hand is extended and about five to seven inches below the surface. As you flex your wrist, your elbow will remain high. Think of pulling yourself over a barrel. This helps with lift and propulsion and serves as a reminder to keep your elbows high.

Finishing the stroke improperly is a common error. We often think that the more strokes we get in the faster we will move through the water. This is not necessarily so. The best swimmers can quickly cover the length of a twenty-five meter pool in only ten to fifteen strokes. One of the reasons for this is that they *finish their stroke*. The back end of the stroke, or the *recovery*, involves pushing the hand as hard and as far as you can to ensure full extension of your arm thus leaving it in a proper position for another stroke.

Now if you understood all that, then you have great visualization skills. The best way to know whether you are following these steps properly is to have someone watch or videotape you. Chip Zempel, a former contributor to *Triathlete* magazine and two-time National Champion marathon swimmer, recommends having someone help you count the time it takes to do ten strokes (i.e., ten complete rotations of the same arm) and note the distance traveled. This is a good exercise because one of the arts of swimming well is to have good stroke efficiency and speed. Zempel found that not only do sprinters have the fastest strokes, but they also manage to cover a greater distance with each stroke. He suggests that an average of eighty-six to eighty-eight strokes per minute for 1,500 meters is good. When racing, however, most swimmers will increase the number of strokes by ten to forty percent over the same distance. Unless you are an accomplished swimmer, focus on the quality of your stroke rather than the speed. One way to incorporate consistent strokes into your workouts is to swim to music with a strong tempo or hum a tune while swimming. This will keep your strokes regular and will help you maintain a consistent speed.

PUTTING IT ALL TOGETHER

- stay flexible by doing regular stretching exercises
- work on the form of your stroke
- practice swim drills for flutter kick, hand entry, body roll and arm movement
- do not overuse swim aids: these should be used for only thirty percent or less of your workout

One instructor had her swimmers imagine themselves swimming through a tube. If their elbows were high and tight, and they made no deep pulls or scissor kicks, they would avoid hitting the tube walls. One well-known swim coach coined the phrase *vessel shaping* which refers to the practice of minimizing the space the body occupies while moving through the water. University of Rochester swim coach Bill Boomer feels that seventy percent of the success in swimming depends on the position of the body in the water and only thirty percent on arm movement. If Boomer is right, swimmers may need to seriously re-evaluate how they train.

We prefer a middle-of-the-road approach. If you work on your form, you should concentrate on being streamlined while propelling your way through the water. Only practice will make this easy. Work on only one or two things at a time. Trying to overcome all your faults at once will only lead to frustration. There are numerous exercises that can isolate the areas of your stroke needing work. For example, you can do kickboard workouts for the legs, use the pull buoys for arm entry and exit workouts, and use one-arm pulls for developing feel and technique. Learning the different strokes will also help your all-round swimming skills and technique. I watch competitive swimmers in training – it is an easy and inexpensive way to learn new tricks and it reinforces the idea that always doing the same stroke does not improve your ability to master the waves. Sticking to the crawl will tend to overdevelop certain muscle groups at the expense of others. This, in turn, increases the risk of injury.

Some of the top pros recommend using the Vasa Trainer® (a swim simulator bench which works on a pulley system) to help with their stroke when access to a pool is not always possible. Six-time Hawaii Ironman winner Dave Scott uses this device. If the price is a little expensive (approximately $800), then you could always purchase some surgical tubing and devise your own pulley system. Some fitness shops carry such pre-made products (approximately $35). The Vasa Trainer® and surgical tubing, among other devices, are helpful for building speed and refining technique.

Pulleys and stretch cords are other inexpensive resistance devices that can be used to improve your stroke and strength. While the pulleys are usually found in gyms, stretch cords can be used at home and they can be used in similar ways. Placing your hands in the loops or paddles, bend your waist and simulate the swim stroke. Be sure to keep elbows high and pull all the way through each stroke. The pulley system provides constant resistance while the stretch cord will provide increased resistance through the pull phase.

Position yourself so that when your arms are forward there is a slight resistance on the cords. Although you can develop your own workout program, it is usually recommended that you do the exercise in sets of twelve to twenty repetitions. Most swim books recommend you do the sets at a slightly faster pace than normal. Remember, you are trying to improve your swim stroke – not be a body builder – so do not think more resistance is always better.

SAMPLE SWIM WORKOUTS FOR SHORT-COURSE TRIATHLON

Pyramids:

$$\frac{\text{I} \cdot 2 \cdot 3 \cdot 4 \cdot 5 \cdot 6 \cdot 5 \cdot 4 \cdot 3 \cdot 2 \cdot \text{I}}{36 \text{ laps in a 25-meter pool}}$$

Allow five to ten seconds of rest between each set of laps. For example, do I lap, rest, do 2 laps, rest, do 3 laps, rest, etc. This helps to build pace and endurance.

Ladders:

$$\frac{100 \cdot 200 \cdot 300 \cdot 400 \cdot 300 \cdot 200 \cdot 100}{64 \text{ laps in a 25-meter pool}}$$

Allow fifteen to thirty seconds of rest between each set of laps. This helps to build endurance and pace.

Half-sprints: Once you have determined your race pace, do five sets of 100 meters each, swimming the first fifty meters of each set at your race pace, then the other fifty meters at an easy pace. It should take roughly four extra minutes to complete 500 meters in this way than it would if you were to go at your race pace throughout. (This is described as "doing race pace plus four minutes"). The purpose of this exercise is to build speed while you are fatigued, in order to improve your stress adaptation.

Broken swims:

$$\frac{11 \cdot 10 \cdot 9 \cdot 8 \cdot 7 \cdot 6 \cdot 5 \cdot 4 \cdot 3 \cdot 2 \cdot 1}{66 \text{ laps in a 25-meter pool}}$$

Allow five to ten seconds of rest between each set. This helps to build pace and endurance.

2,000 meters: Divide this swim into four groups of twenty laps each, with a one-minute rest in between. This helps to build endurance. Try to maintain a consistent pace.

Fartlek: Vary the pace according to your whim. This helps to build pace.

TWO SAMPLE SWIM WORKOUTS

FIRST WORKOUT

1. Warm up with an easy 400 meters.

2. Using a kick board and pull buoy, swim 12 × 75 m (go at race pace plus 4–5 minutes – see Half-sprints above).
   - First 75 m is 50 m pull, 25 m kick
   - Second 75 m is 25 m kick, 50 m pull
   - Third 75 m is 50 m kick, 25 m pull
   - Fourth 75 m is 25 m pull, 50 m kick
   - Repeat the entire cycle three times (Total = 900 m)

3. Swim 10 × 50 m at a moderate pace that makes you work but does not cause undue stress.

- ► two × 50 m breathing every 2 strokes
- ► two × 50 m breathing every 3 strokes
- ► two × 50 m breathing every 5 strokes
- ► two × 50 m breathing every 6 strokes
- ► two × 50 m breathing every 8 strokes (Total = 500 m)

4. Swim 20 × 25 meters at just below race pace.
   - ► Divide into four sets of 25 m in which you decrease the amount of breathing in each set. Start with five breaths per 25 m then decrease to four, three, two and one breath before repeating the cycle (total = 500 m).

5. Easy backstroke or breaststroke (100 m).

6. Swim 10 × 25 m, gradually decreasing the intensity: swim laps 1–3 hard, laps 4–7 moderate and laps 7–9 easy. Swim at race pace plus 3–4 minutes. Do the tenth flat out (total = 250 m).

7. Cool down (250 m).

   Total = 2,900 meters

SECOND WORKOUT

1. Warm-up with an easy 400 m.

2. Using a flutter board, swim 10 × 25 m alternating easy and hard pace.

3. Using a flutter board, swim 20 × 25 m kick at race pace.

4. Swim 10 × 25 m alternating easy and hard pace.

5. Using a pull buoy, swim 20 × 25 m arm pull at race pace plus 3 minutes.

6. Swim 10 × 25 m alternating easy and hard pace.

7. Swim 100 m using only your legs.

8. Using a pull buoy, swim 2 × 100 m using your arms only at race pace plus three minutes. Concentrate on form and technique.

9. Swim 400 m timed. Record your time for future comparison.

10. Swim 150 m at an easy pace to cool down.

    Total = 3,000 meters

GETTING AROUND IN THE WATER

There is a big difference between swimming in a pool and swimming in open water. The following tips and observations are intended for less experienced swimmers.

THE POOL

One of the most significant changes to swimming pools in recent years has been the introduction of saline (salt) solution pools. In the past, most pools were chlorinated for sanitary purposes but this often wrought havoc on the skin and hair of regular swimmers. Many competitive swimmers can recount stories of their hair turning green or falling out, and skin cracking because of the bleaching and dehydrating effect of the chlorine. Fortunately, many pools have now converted to salt water which is less harsh on the body and the environment. An added benefit of saline water is that you get better buoyancy.

Pools are excellent for controlled workouts because you can accurately measure the distance and time of each session. The sample swim workouts presented above are designed to be done in a pool. In addition to the different types of swim workouts you can do, the safe confines of a pool provide a great setting for learning bilateral breathing and practicing drafting. These are two important elements of open-water swimming and racing.

Drafting is of great value in swimming, in cycling, speed skating, cross-country skiing and most sports where speed is important. While drafting on the bike is generally illegal in most triathlons (but not regular cycle races), it is not illegal in the swim. Moving through the water creates considerable resistance and in drafting, you swim directly behind someone thereby allowing them to break the resistance so you can swim faster. Just be sure not to run into the person ahead of you and be sure that they know how to swim a straight line! You might even want to consider teaming up with someone and taking turns "pulling." (This strategy is used by cyclists to help maintain high speeds.) As the one team swimmer appears to let up, the other moves to the front and swims hard for a while.

OPEN-WATER SWIMMING

If you are going to participate in a triathlon you will almost certainly have to swim in open water. Other than playing in lakes or rivers as kids, many of us never really swam in open water. It can be very intimidating. I know several people who swam races in pools but felt uncomfortable in open water. Many swimmers are uneasy when they cannot see the bottom or judge how deep the water is, and often they fear an encounter with an "open-water creature."

If you are not used to swimming in open water but wish to give it a try then seek relatively calm, familiar and warm water. It is also helpful to seek shallow water and stay close to shore, just in case you need to stop. In addition, it is wise to have someone accompany you either in the water or on some flotation device – preferably one that does not have a motor. Smelling gas fumes while swimming is not pleasant.

Another aspect of open-water swimming in a race is the mass start. Although it is an impressive sound at water level to hear hundreds of arms churning up the water, the fear of being kicked, or someone crawling right over you can be enough to stop many from even attempting the waters. It is important to seed (place) yourself according to your ability. When in doubt go toward the back.

A further challenge of open-water swimming is keeping yourself headed in a straight line. Pool swimming is easy. Often without knowing it, you correct your stroke by following the lines at the bottom of the pool. In open water there are no guides. Karen is notorious for drifting to the right. We figure she usually gets twice the workout when we are at the lake. Fortunately, there are simple ways to correct the tendency to pull left or right.

In a race you can use the guide boats to steer you or you can keep an eye on the shoreline – assuming it is straight. It is better to lift your head every few strokes and look forward. The most effective way to do this is to have your head follow your arm as you complete a recovery stoke. An additional technique is to learn bilateral breathing, that is, breathing on both sides. Distance swimmers usually alternate every third stroke. In this way you can look out from both sides as well as look forward from time to time. Failing all else, you can temporarily switch to the breast-stroke in order to look around and make sure you are on track. When you are swimming in a large group this can make the difference between running into people and having a strong and comfortable swim. I have even seen swimmers roll over into a backstroke to look behind them to gauge the competition.

THE WETSUIT

In northern climates we are often subjected to cool, if not cold, water conditions. It is not uncommon to race in water with a temperature hovering in the low sixties. And until recently, the use of wetsuits was a controversial issue, and to some extent it still is.

Officially, the International Triathlon Union (ITU) has ruled that if the water is over 72°F (22°C) wetsuits are not allowed. However, there have been several incidents over the past few years where race officials have been criticized for claiming the water to be warmer than it was. The problem is that while wet-suits have been proven to cut swimming times by an average of fifty-one seconds per 1,000 meters, the rules are still not always fairly applied as some races use rather questionable methods of measuring water temperature.

Therefore, unless you are told otherwise, wear a wetsuit so long as you're not swimming in bath water. A recent survey conducted in Australia found that one hundred percent of the elite triathletes used wetsuits when permitted as did over eighty percent of the non-elite athletes. Swimmers should always be wary of cool water because of the risk of hypothermia which may prevent you from continuing or seriously slow you down. A wetsuit will allow you to save time in the swim and the extra time required to take off a wetsuit is negligible considering most of your competitors will be doing the same.

Until the controversy is settled, enjoy the extra speed and comfort. With wetsuit technology changing each year, it is difficult to recommend one suit over another. The best rule of thumb is to test them yourself. Full wetsuits (long legs and arms) can be too restrictive, shortened legs make for quick removal, and cutout sleeves make arm turnover easier.

In the meantime, the ITU and other governing bodies might want to pay attention to Dr. Gary Shinn's (Chairman of the Medical Committee Triathlon of Australia) recommendation. He recommends all professional divisions and elite athletes under the age of 35 not be allowed to wear wetsuits when the water temperature is at or above 71.6°F (22°C). All others should be allowed to choose regardless of water temperature. Wetsuits, says Shinn, have become a mainstay in triathlons and they should be used strictly in the interest of safety.

As you work on your swimming, you should also focus on your cycling technique. So let us move on.

Chapter 6

Cycling

Although most of us know how to ride a bicycle, riding fast and well takes knowledge and practice. In this chapter we will review the essential elements of this sport which, if followed, will make you a more efficient cyclist and better prepared to race.

· The faster your cycling cadence, the more your legs become conditioned to pumping faster and the more speed you will have when running.

· You will only cycle at your potential if you are comfortable on your bike.

· If you can reduce your wind resistance, you can go faster with the same energy output.

CUSTOM FITTING

The cycling portion of a triathlon takes the greatest amount of time. For an Ironman race you can spend five or more hours in the saddle while for a short course you might spend an hour on your bike. Regardless of the event, you will not enjoy the ride, nor will you cycle at your potential unless you feel comfortable on your bike. Poor fitting can lead to a number of common cycling ailments, such as:

▸ saddle soreness

▸ lower back pain

▸ knee strain

▸ numbness in the feet

▸ numbness in the crotch

- tightness in the shoulders and neck

- sore palms

Proper bike fitting is essential for a comfortable ride. In addition, you will find that your fitness is influenced by the way you and your bike fit together. Therefore, it is worth spending time on how your bike fits. Unless you have the time and inclination to do your own fitting, go to a reputable cycle shop. In the meantime, here are some basic pointers.

FRAME SIZE AND FORM FITTING

Straddle your bike in your bare feet. You should be able to put your fist between the top tube and your crotch. If you are riding a suspension/beam bike (a bike in which the top tube and down tubes are not joined, and where the seat is attached to the top tube), you will not be able to apply the same test because of the angle of the beam. In this case you need to refer to the frame size guidelines sidebar below. Also, given that these bikes allow you to adjust the height and angle of the beam and the position of the saddle, it is a simple matter of experimentation to find the ideal fit. John Howard, a former Ironman winner and holder of numerous cycling records, recommends smaller frames as they tend to be stronger and lighter and they handle better than larger ones.

In *The Complete Book of Cycling*, Greg LeMond (three-time Tour de France winner) offers a more scientific formula for calculating frame size. Take your inseam and then multiply that figure by .65. For example, my inseam is approximately 91 cm. Using LeMond's formula, 91 cm × .65 = 59.15. My frame (60 cm) fits both the basic formula given above and LeMond's calculation. Some have suggested LeMond's calculations may yield a slightly larger frame than is ideal. On the other hand, Van de Plas' method involves subtracting 10.5 inches/26.5 cm from your inseam. This measurement may yield a slightly undersized frame.

In short, any sizing based on inseam measurement is subject to some limitations. This is because the sizing does not take into account the torso length, arm length, and shoulder width. Usually only a custom builder will look at the whole body and how it should be matched to a bike.

Once you have determined your ideal frame size, you can then test for form fit, that is, how the stem length and seat height fits your body. Get someone to hold the bike while you sit in the saddle and place your hands on the brake hoods. How do you feel? Too stretched out? Too cramped? Or relaxed? Look at some pictures of top cyclists on their bikes and then look at yourself in the mirror – how do you compare? Form fit is somewhat individual, but the key is to feel relaxed while in a normal riding position. It is best to get yourself professionally fitted by someone who will also pay attention to your cycling needs.

Since some of you may not have access to such shops, the following tips can be helpful when you are buying a new bike. Keep in mind how much time you would like, or hope, to spend on your two-wheel investment. If you ride your bike for six hours or more a week you are likely to appreciate a good fit. If your bike isn't right for your body, it is like having a pair of shoes either too small or too big and then having to stand on your feet all day. Professional riders are extremely choosy.

Take the time to experiment with the following guidelines. Make any changes such as handlebar or seat adjustments gradually and allow a week or two before you make any additional changes. This will allow your body to adapt comfortably to even the most subtle adjustment. It is not uncommon to hear neophytes complain about lower back pain after adding aero bars to their frame. The increased extension of the lower back adds stress which can be painful.

▸ When resting on the drops of the handle bars you should not see the front hub. If you do, the handlebar stem and/or top tube is either too short or too long or the actual frame may be incorrect for you. The handle/aero bars should be as wide apart as your shoulders to allow for proper breathing, especially when climbing. If you look down through the top of the handlebar stem with your hands on the brake hoods the front axle should appear approximately 5 cm above the handlebar stem.

► Determining the height of the seat, although easily done, is critical for attaining maximum leg torque. Get someone to support you or use a stationary wind trainer to keep your bike stable. Then mount your bike in shoeless feet. Adjust the pedals so that they are at 12 and 6 o'clock (straight up and down). In this position the heel of your extended leg should just touch the pedal. Adjust your seat height as required. If your seat is too high you will likely experience lower back pain and quadricep fatigue and if it is too low, you will likely feel quadricep fatigue, decreased power and pain under the kneecap from excess strain on the knee.

► Determining the height of the seat, although easily done, is critical for attaining maximum leg torque. If you have followed the above point you should be fine.

► With the pedals at 3 and 9 o'clock (horizontal), you should be able to grasp the top tube with your knees. If not, the frame will be either too big or too small or the seat will be set at the wrong height. Common sense will tell which is the case.

► A final indicator that you have the right frame size is that whatever saddle height you set, your hips do not rock side to side when you pedal. If they do, your seat is too high.

WHAT'S IN A FRAME?

If you have ever observed a bike race or walked into a quality bike shop, you will no doubt realize that the cycling industry has come a long way from the days when we all rode stock bikes from our local department store. One of the popular cycling magazines reported that the top racing bikes in 1996 weighed nearly twenty-five percent less than they did in the mid-1980s. Fully accessorized racing bikes can weigh well under eighteen pounds. Today virtually no part of the bike has not been revolutionized – all in the name of performance! Bikes have become lighter, stiffer and more costly. The stiffer the frame, the more power that is transmitted from the pedals to forward motion as opposed to being lost in a frame that flexes too much. One of the challenges for bike builders is to make a bike that is light and stiff, yet also durable and "sensitive" enough to provide a comfortable ride. We will review the main frame materials and suggest that you make a decision based first on the results of your test rides, and then on cost.

FRAME SIZE GUIDELINES

HEIGHT	·	FRAME SIZE
< 160 cm	►	50 cm
160–164 cm	►	52 cm
165–174 cm	►	55 cm
175–180 cm	►	58 cm
> 180 cm	►	61 cm

STEEL CHROME-MOLY

The oldest and most common bicycle building material is steel. Steel is usually cheaper, more durable and easier to repair than other materials. Virtually all grades of steel include one or more small additions of titanium, vanadium, copper and columbium to make the bike lighter while still maintaining its strength.

While steel frames tend to be heavier than other frames, it is the rolling or moving weight which is most critical. Therefore, if you like the look and feel of a steel frame then you can still minimize overall weight by using the money you save to buy lightweight wheels, cranks, freewheel, pedals and pulleys.

ALUMINUM

Companies like Cannondale and Klein have cut out a very nice niche in the bicycle market with their aluminum frames. When they first appeared, most conventional cyclists laughed at the oversize tubing and bulkiness of these bikes. However, they often weighed less (aluminum is about one-third as dense as steel) than steel frames, offered comparable stiffness and in some cases a slightly softer ride.

Aluminum and its various alloys are highly resistant to corrosion, making it a favorite in damp climates. Furthermore, it is generally easier to weld than specialized steel tubing and so production costs are lower. Many companies use combinations of aluminum and composite materials to add strength and reduce weight. Vitus bikes were among the first to experiment successfully with such frames.

TITANIUM

Titanium is one of the most resilient metals, it will not corrode, it looks hot and it has a higher strength to weight ratio than steel – but it is lighter by about forty-five percent. As with aluminum frames, however, titanium frames tend to be slightly oversized in order to maximize their strength to weight ratio. The metal is also mixed with aluminum and vanadium to enhance strength and performance. The major drawback of these frames is still their cost and it is likely most people will only be dreaming about them for a long time to come.

COMPOSITE MATERIAL

Just as the term suggests, composite frames are made from a combination of materials. Typically they involve kevlar, graphite, ceramic and boron. These materials can be woven together to build esthetic and radical looking frames. They can be welded, glued and even built as a complete frame – referred to as a *monoque* frame. These tend to be the most expensive frames on the market and, unless money is no object and weight or image is important, you will prefer to explore other frame materials. Be aware that repairs on composite frames can be difficult and expensive.

Since your frame is the most important element of your bike, you should carefully consider cost, durability, weight, reliability and performance. A quality frame can last many years.

GO AERODYNAMIC AND BE EFFICIENT

At 20 m.p.h. (32 km per hour), a rider on a conventional bike can displace about 1,000 pounds (450 kg) of air per minute. This type of effort consumes ninety percent of the rider's energy. To get up to 26 m.p.h. (42 km per hour), however, would require twice the output! The speed record for a conventional bike is just over 30 m.p.h. (48 km per hour) while for an aerodynamically designed bike, the record is 47 m.p.h. (76 km per hour). The faster you move, however, the greater the drag (i.e., wind resistance) and the more energy is required to maintain the same speed. Therefore, if you can reduce your wind resistance you can go faster with the same energy output. In the 1994 Hawaii Ironman, it was said that Ken Glah, who had the fastest cycling time, was able to reach such great speeds because he had spent time in a wind tunnel fine-tuning his aerodynamic position. The result of this training was that he was able to save about twenty minutes over the 112-mile (180-km) course!

Here are some hot tips to help you get the most speed when cycling.

▸ *Low and Narrow.* Your cycling position can dramatically affect your speed – the idea is to be as aerodynamic as possible. (And since your bike only accounts for thirty to forty-nine percent of the total aerodynamic drag, the primary culprit is *you*!) Experts agree that when it comes to positioning your body, you should get low and narrow. This generally involves keeping a flat back and putting your shoulder height below your hip height – so long as you are still able to pedal with your knees held in. Keep your elbows as close together as is practically possible. This forces you to roll your shoulders in and form a tuck position which allows the air to flow around your body. Set your bike up on a stationary windtrainer and experiment with these positions.

▶ *Head Tilt.* Because you should always wear a helmet when cycling, it is best to hold your head up slightly. This will maximize the aerodynamic qualities of your helmet. You should be able to see comfortably about fifteen feet ahead of you.

▶ *Arm Angle.* Cycling expert Boone Lennon suggests that the cant of your arm should be somewhere between horizontal and a 30-degree tilt. (Ken Glah's ideal forearm tilt is 15 degrees combined with his upper arms extended to 45 degrees). Test yourself for efficiency and comfort. Most importantly, allow your body time to adjust to any positioning changes, otherwise you are simply inviting injury.

If you want to race in the aero position, you must practice training in the aero position. Failure to do so may cause back problems in a race and you are not likely to get the same power transfer because your body is not yet used to performing in the different position.

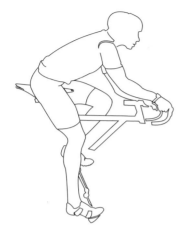

THE TRADITIONAL CYCLING
POSITION. NOTE THE OPEN
CHEST — GREAT WIND
RESISTANCE!

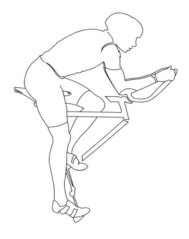

THE UNDESIRABLE CYCLING
POSITION. THE LEGS ARE OVEREX-
TENDED, THE BACK IS CURLED AND
THE POSITION IS UPRIGHT.

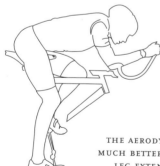

THE AERODYNAMIC CYCLING POSITION. AH!
MUCH BETTER. FLAT BACK, LOW PROFILE, GOOD
LEG EXTENSION AND BALANCED WEIGHT
DISTRIBUTION OVER THE BAR.

GEARS AND GEARING

One of the most frequently overlooked aspects of becoming a good cyclist is mastering the gears. Learning proper gearing can result in big rewards while improper gearing will (sooner or later) be felt in the legs.

Assuming you have some type of standard road bike, you will have two chain rings in the front – a big and a small one. On the rear wheel you will have a series of sprockets (rear chain rings) that are arranged from the smallest on the outside to the largest on the inside. Together these sprockets are referred to as a "cog set" or "freewheel."

In order to ride efficiently, you need to learn how many teeth each of the rings in the front has (usually 52 and 42) as well as the number in the back (usually 12 through 21). Cyclists will often say things like, "I had to use 42 × 18 to climb that big hill," or on the flats, "I was pushing "52 × 12." The first number always refers to the front chain ring while the second number refers the rear cog being used.

The real challenge comes from knowing how to properly use your gears and which ones to buy. Since the rear clusters are cheaper to replace than the front rings you may want to experiment with different combinations. A typical rear nine-speed cluster might include 12·13·14·15·16·17·18·20·23. The single increments allow the rider to fine-tune the power phase of their ride while the upper gears (e.g., 18, 20 and 23), sometimes referred to as "granny" or "bail-out" gears, are used when speed is no longer an issue, but when finishing the ride or making it up a hill is.

If you have some type of cycle computer that includes a cadence indicator then you can use it to gauge which gearing combination you should be using. Whether going uphill, downhill, into the wind or with the wind, you should maintain a cadence between 80 and 100 r.p.m. With experience you will learn to adjust your gearing so as to maintain good cadence. As stated earlier, maintaining proper cadence will help to ensure that you are not overloading your knees or placing undue stress on your lower back. To fine-tune your gearing even more, wear a heart-rate monitor and pay attention to how different gearing combinations can help to keep your heart rate down while still maintaining desired speed. As there is no magic formula, this is something you can experiment with. Cycling aids such as the Computrainer® include a spin indicator which provides visual feedback on how efficiently you are pedaling at different speeds and with different gearing combinations. Yes, it can get all very scientific and technical, but if you learn the fundamentals, you can then refine your cycling as you become more in-tune with your bike.

You could spend a lot of time studying gear ratios and trying to figure out if you have any duplication of gears. Most bike shops, however, will fix you up with a reliable front-rear configuration that will meet most, if not all, your needs. If you tell them what kind of course you'll be racing on, they might recommend changing a few of the cogs. While most store-bought bikes come all set up, you might want to learn about gear ratios in order to tailor your gearing to specific race and riding conditions. For example, when I raced a relatively flat course I used a rear cluster that had no granny gears. Instead, the freewheel might include a range from 11–17 (I use to use a seven-speed cluster then) with 49 and 55 front chain rings. For a demanding course such as Ironman Canada, I would have a 23 for the big hills and strong winds. For my front chain rings I would switch to 42 and 53. If you decide to tinker with your freewheel and chain rings you should ensure you have a combination that ensures an optimum range of gears. This is especially important now that nine-speed cog sets are standard and ten-speed sets are also available.

WHEELS

Your wheels create wind resistance. Aside from the actual rolling weight, the number and type of spokes, rim type, tire type, tire pressure and wheel size all contribute to aerodynamic drag.

Much has been written about which wheels are the fastest and strongest. Rather than present and analyze all the data here, let's prioritize the options. A good deep-rim front wheel with the least number of radial-patterned, bladed spokes should be your first choice. The rear wheel should be a disk or deep-rim wheel with a spoke pattern that allows for strength but does not seriously compromise the overall aerodynamic qualities of the wheel. Since the rear wheel is subjected to a greater amount of stress than the front wheel, consider a rear wheel that has a greater number of spokes. Spokes on the inside (cog side) should have some type of cross-over pattern for strength; the outside spokes can be radial. Your wheel configuration should be dictated by your weight, riding style and the terrain.

As for the spoke industry, it is generally agreed that bladed spokes are faster than rounded ones. It is now possible, however, to buy elliptic carbon fiber spokes which, in addition to being lighter, also generate less drag.

Finally, depending on your choice, you can pay as little as CDN$600 for a set of wheels which have aero rims, low spoke configuration and weigh a scant 1,895 grams. On the other hand, you can pay up to CDN$2,000 for high-tech composite wheels. Top-of-the-line wheels can weigh as little as 1,949 grams. They are made of a carbon composite and have deep rims.

If you start to get into tri spokes and solid disk wheels, the cost can literally double or triple. You will need to decide the cost benefit. Personally, I prefer to use the less expensive aero wheels and put the money I saved into other drag-reduction components.

"Given similar structural and aerodynamic characteristics, a lighter wheel is always faster." (*Triathlete*). Smaller wheels accelerate faster and are lighter, but may generate a little more turbulence (the wind resistance created by air movement around the tires). Seven-time Ironwoman winner Paula Newby-Fraser has used a 24-inch wheel in Hawaii while many other top triathletes use the less radical 26-inch wheels. Since most top-of-the-line manufacturers build frames for both 26-inch (mountain bike) and 700c (road bike) wheels, it would appear once again that you should consider cost, practicality and finally test ride them before making any major purchase.

Your tires should be inflated to the recommended pressure. This will reduce rolling resistance. Buy quality tires which are rated for 110–170 p.s.i. There are several good brand names on the market which differ according to weight, width and durability. Your weight and the condition of the course should dictate which tire and which width to go for. The worse the road conditions, the heavier and wider the tire required, and it often helps to have slightly *less* than the recommended air pressure when the roads are bad. This will help your tires maintain better contact with the road. You lose speed anytime there is insufficient contact between road and tire. The advantages of using narrow, lightweight tires on rough roads can be lost if you get a flat or even if your bike is constantly bouncing around. Therefore, know the course and the conditions, and plan accordingly.

CLOTHING

The special gear worn by cyclists also deserves some consideration. There are plenty of fabrics and garments available to improve the comfort of your ride. Here are a few remarks on the basic elements of the cyclist's wardrobe.

▶ Cycling shorts are specially designed to maximize your comfort while in the saddle. They usually have some type of padding in the crotch. There are even shorts whose padded sections are cut specifically to fit men, and others cut just for women. These will be labeled accordingly.

▸ The jerseys are usually made of a special material that permits cooling and wicks sweat away from the body. They also tend to have two or three pockets on the back in which to place food, extra riding gear, tools, or other small and relatively light objects.

▸ Shaved legs, aside from vanity, make wounds easier to clean should you crash.

▸ Helmets are a safety necessity for anyone who wants to ride – regardless of whether you are in an urban or rural setting.

▸ Cycling gloves are specially designed to increase hand comfort and reduce road shock.

▸ Ever notice cyclists with those funny boot covers? When you can travel at high speed, your feet can get considerably cooler than you might think. During cool or rainy days, booties can add a significant degree of comfort. And if your feet get too warm, just take them off and stick them in one of the back panels of your jersey. Some neoprene versions on the market are excellent at keeping your feet warm and dry. Be sure that the underside will fit the type of pedal system you have.

Optional equipment includes an extra bike just for training during inclement weather, extra cycling shoes, a cycling jersey which has convenient carrying pockets in the back, cycling gloves, an air pump, sunglasses, aero-type bars, disk wheels, a repair kit (with a spare tube, tire, tire remover, multipurpose wrench and spoke adjustment key).

Cycle computers are another piece of equipment you should consider having. They provide a wealth of information and are excellent motivating tools. Depending on the model, they can tell you the distance you have traveled, your average speed, actual speed, travel time and cadence. Some models are equipped

with altitude meters while others have built-in heart-rate monitors and backlights.

ANSWERS TO COMMONLY-ASKED QUESTIONS

▸ *Should I use clincher or tubular tires?* Tubulars (the type of tire
you glue onto the rim) cost more but some claim they provide
a smoother ride. They are usually lighter, more expensive,
more responsive and they are able to handle higher pressure.
Another advantage of tubulars is that should you get a flat in
the last few kilometers of the course, you can ride a tubular or
"sew-up" with some basic comfort while a clincher will wobble
around uncontrollably making any type of riding less than
comfortable or safe. Also, while clinchers may be cheaper, they
generally take more time to replace than sew-ups. On the flip
side, unless you have sufficient glue remaining on your rim
after replacing a flat, sew-ups are less reliable when cornering.
The key is to know the course conditions and what your objectives are. For training I use clinchers but for racing I switch to
tubulars.

▸ *What pedals should I use?* There are well over a dozen different
systems for securing your feet to the pedals. Assuming you no
longer use the old toe strap or rat-trap system, the main choice
today is between a fixed or foot float pedal system. Fixed pedals do not allow any foot movement, while foot float pedals
allow your foot to move several degrees laterally. The objective
is to allow the foot and knee to move more naturally and
thereby reduce any unnecessary stress on the ligaments. If
you have any knee problems, a foot float pedal might be the
answer for you. There are other models on the market and
most of the major brands produce a range of pedals whose
weight and features vary. Pedals also range widely in price
from around CDN$60 for low-end models to over CDN$350 for
a set of top-of-the-line pedals. Most of the teams in the 1996

Tour de France used some type of foot float pedal, while track specialists tend to prefer the fixed pedal system. These allow the maximum transfer of power, hence greater speed.

An often ignored aspect of pedal system is the proximity of the spindle or axis of the pedal to your foot. The closer the axle is to your foot, the greater the transfer of energy will be to the pedal. Today, a number of shoe and pedal combinations allow you to control the amount of foot flotation and the tension controlling your foot release. The shoe-pedal set-up allows your foot to be closer to the center point of the axle thus providing a superior feel and better road clearance when cornering.

One of "hottest" new systems on the pedal market is the *transition pedal system*. Currently, there are three such systems available. Ideal for multisport events, these are platform systems which enable you to wear your running shoes while cycling. They are relatively light, have an adjustable heel gripper to fit your shoe size, a toe cage and a fastening strap to keep you locked in. Many of the top triathlon and duathlon professionals have used this new concept successfully in short races. They range in weight from about 210 to 238 grams and cost between CDN$60 and CDN$99. Some systems require cleat adapters. Unless you are a duathlete, transition pedal systems are probably not a prudent choice. A growing number of companies are producing multipurpose shoes which have a built-in cleat system that also allows you to walk around with a reasonable degree of comfort. While not practical for racing, they make fine training shoes.

▸ *What features should I look for in cycling shoes?* Proper shoes are important for comfort and pedaling technique. Most triathletes today use single- or double-velcro fastening shoes for easy entry and exit during a race. In addition to basic comfort, you might also want to consider the weight of the shoe – as usual, less is better.

It is always a good idea to make sure any shoe inserts you use are removable. Some companies make inserts which will fit your cycling shoes. They come in different densities and can be molded to correct orthopedic problems. Having used molded orthotics for over a decade without incurring any knee or leg injury, I swear by them. Most active people can probably benefit from orthotic inserts.

▸ *How do I determine the ideal crank for me?* Crank arms are subjected to incredible amounts of force and torque, especially during climbing or sprinting. Therefore you will want very stiff cranks to ensure that all that power is used for forward motion. While light cranks are desirable, they do not offer as much strength as the heavier ones. Longer crank arms enable you to generate more power, though not without trade-offs. Longer cranks are harder on your knees and leg muscles, and tend to lower the number of revolutions per minute you make. The ideal length for your cranks will depend on your muscle strength, level of conditioning and leg length. Use Table 6.1 as a general guideline when buying cranks.

Table 6.1 GENERAL GUIDELINE FOR DETERMINING CRANK LENGTH

INSEAM LENGTH (INCHES)	PRE-SEASON (mm)	RACE-SEASON (mm)	CHAIN RING SIZE (NUMBER OF TEETH)
25	165.0	167.5	52
26–28	167.5	170.0	52
29–33	170.0	172.0	52, 53
34–36	172.5	175.0	53, 54
37–40	175.0	177.5–180.0	54, 55, 56

The rationale for a shorter pre-season crank length is that it reduces stress on your legs and enables you to spin. Then, when you switch to the pre-race-season cranks, you can maintain the same cadence but generate more power and speed . . . that's smart training!

5. *What should I know about seats?* A wide variety of saddles on the market claim to have ergonomic advantages. These advantages include a light, aerodynamic design, special rail material that reduces weight and absorbs road shock, and built-in suspension pads under the seat. Again, you pay a price for all the special features but, unless you are comfortable in the saddle, gadgets mean nothing. Ask to test ride a saddle for a few hours or days, if possible.

Men will need to pay attention to their seat and riding positions. If the seat nose or your position is too high, you may develop numbness in a sensitive area. This is not uncommon and some subtle adjustments can minimize this unwelcome feeling (or lack thereof). John Howard recommends lowering the seat nose two to three degrees for added comfort. This also places you in a more aggressive position, and gives you a more powerful pelvic tilt. This subtle adjustment will also increase the power of your biggest muscles, the hamstrings and gluts.

If you want to read more about the seat height, seat positioning and other technical elements, see Edmund Burke's book *Science of Cycling.*

DESIGNED FOR WOMEN

In recent years, the cycling industry has begun to build bikes and cycling equipment that take into account the anatomical differences between men and women. For example, women's frames have shorter top tubes, and women's saddles are specially designed to relieve pressure. A number of companies are even building cycling shoes with a stiff midsole built on a women's last (the molded form that gives the shoe its shape and structure). It is even possible to get cycling shorts for pregnant women. One of the first manufacturers to design cycles, equipment and clothes specifically for women and one of the leaders in the industry is Georgina Terry.

YOU STILL NEED TO TRAIN

Cycling involves endurance, speed and strength. Your training program should include all these aspects with extra attention given to your weaknesses. Table 6.2 offers a small sampling of indoor workouts you can do when the weather is inclement. If done properly, you may even be able to get better quality workouts on your stationary wind trainer. For example, Jeff Devlin who finished third in Hawaii in 1994 and Ken Glah who had the fastest bike split in the 1994 Hawaii Ironman, spent most of their winter months on stationary wind trainers. If time is limited you might want to consider this option. Although it is wonderful to get outdoors and train, sometimes the weather and your schedule make it impossible to get in a good open-air workout. Indoor riding workouts can be just as specialized as outdoor ones, and they can always be done at your convenience. Table 6.2 shows a range of workouts covering everything from developing basic speed, all-round fitness and an efficient riding form. These workouts complement all the essential elements of becoming a better rider.

Note: Each stationary wind trainer has its own resistance, so it is better to rely on your heart rate and cadence (r.p.m.) as your guide to proper gearing.

Table 6.2 INDOOR RIDING WORKOUTS

KEY: Your front chain ring usually has three rings while your rear cog will have a set of rings ranging in size and number of teeth. In the first workout, 42 refers to one of the front cogs; "x" refers to the combination of a front cog with a rear cog. BR refers to the big front ring while SR refers to the smaller of the front rings. The abbreviation r.p.m. refers to revolutions per minute. If you have a cycle computer it may have a cadence/ r.p.m. function on it. AT is your anaerobic threshold (60–75% of your maximum heart rate).

PURPOSE	WARM-UP	WORK	COOL DOWN
develop speed	5 min each 42 × 19,19,17,15	10–20 reps • 15 sec hard • 45 sec easy	3 min each 42 × 15,17,19
develop recovery	same	5–25 reps • 1 min at 90–100+ r.p.m. • spin out after until HR is 60% AT	same
develop power	same	3–8 reps BR • at 90 r.p.m. • 2–3 min recovery between	same
all-round fitness	same	• 3 min 90 r.p.m. with 3×20 sec all out • 3 × 1 min 100–120 r.p.m. all out • 3 × 2 min at 85% AT hold 100 r.p.m.	same
active recovery		60–70% effort … sustained effort watching your favorite triathlon video, show, etc. Duration: 45–75 minutes.	
develop endurance	45 min to 2 hr of anything else … cross-country skiing/roller blading	Do any of the above relatively soon after!	same
teaches smooth & powerful pedaling	same	4–8 reps • 6 × 30 sec alternating one-leg spins. (Place other leg on chair.) • 30–40 sec recovery Build up to 3–5 min per leg with 2–3 min recovery.	same

Note: Most of these workouts will take less than one hour but if done correctly will offer excellent rewards when you can ride outdoors again. Remember these are merely samples; think about your objective and *play*. Another option is to use a SuperNintendo® video unit that connects your stationary cycle to your television. The Nintendo® software has numerous on-screen programs and gives you the option of programming your own course. The unit allows you to watch yourself race against another rider on-screen or, if you have the software, you can race against a friend in another town or country. In addition to being able to design your own program, you can even draft a pacer, or use the SpinScan® program to analyze pedal efficiency and leg power split. Not only is the Nintendo Unit highly motivating and fun, but it is an effective and safe training system.

CYCLING-SPECIFIC STRENGTH TRAINING WORKOUTS

Cycling requires strong legs and a strong back. The following two workouts have been designed to increase strength in your legs and back and should be incorporated into your strength training program. When doing the leg workouts, the *down* phase means you move into the position (e.g., lunge or dead lift) while the *up* phase means you return to your normal stance.

- General preparation phase: 1 second down – 1 second up
- Strength phase: 2 seconds down – 2 seconds up
- Power phase: 3 seconds down – 1 second up

Remember: your kneecap should never pass beyond the ball of your foot during the lunge exercise. Do not hyperextend your knees during straight leg dead lifts.

Warm up and stretch before, between and after each session. If you are unfamiliar with any of the exercises, most of them can be found in *Getting Stronger* by Bill Pearl and Gary Moran. Please note that these are only general descriptions of the strength-training exercises and you should only try these with the supervision and guidance of a professional physiologist or weight-trainer.

WORKOUT 1

- *Lunges – standing.* Holding dumbbells in each hand, step forward (this is called lunging). Your forward leg should not bend more than ninety degrees. Good for balance, gluts (buttocks), hamstrings and quadriceps.

▶ *Straight leg dead lifts.* This can be done with a barbell or dumb-bells. With feet about eight inches apart, reach down and grasp the weights. Then with legs straightened, back straight, head up and elbows locked, straighten up. Keeping your legs straight, lower the weight. Good for gluts, thighs and lower back.

▶ *Inclined leg press.* Using an inclined leg press machine, place your feet about ten cm apart and lower the weight so your knees are at a ninety degree angle – no more. Then straighten your legs. Most machines have a safety bar – use it. Many inclined benches also have a back adjustment. The lower it is set, the greater the range of motion demanded of the body. Good for quads, gluts and lower back.

▶ *Hack squat.* With this machine you will lift weight that rests on your shoulders. Your back is supported by a pad. When ready, release the safety bar and perform squats until your legs are at a ninety degree angle. Keep back straight and head up. This is good for your upper thighs.

▶ *Leg extension* (optional). Here you use a machine where you sit with your forefoot under a padded bar and then lift the bar upwards with your leg. This is good for strengthening your thighs.

WORKOUT 2

▶ *Vertical leg press and horizontal leg press.* Most gyms have both these machines. On the vertical leg press machine you lift the weight upward while on the horizontal leg press you are in a semi-reclined position and push your leg outward. Both machines and exercises are good for hamstrings and quadri-ceps as well as for building power.

▶ *Seated hamstring.* Some machines involve sitting down and using your heels pull a bar back under you, while other machines require you to lay down over a bench and pull a bar up toward your backside.

▸ *Calf raises.* There are a wide variety of machines for doing calf raises. Essentially they all involve working the calf muscle by having you raise a weight using your calves independently or together. Good for calf muscles and ankle flexion.

RIDING TIPS

1. Getting from the start to the finish line in the shortest period of time is the name of the game. To do so, find your optimum cadence in training (between 80–110 r.p.m. – check your bike speed against your heart rate and your general state of well-being after your ride). Practice staying in the saddle as much as possible, even on the hills. Standing on your pedals requires considerably more energy than riding seated. Use proper gears and cadence to keep yourself in the saddle.

2. Try to maintain a cadence between 80 and 110 r.p.m. On really steep grades try to keep it above 70 r.p.m. (If you ride a beam system then your cadence is likely to drop slightly by 5–10 r.p.m.). Maintaining a proper cadence will ensure that you are not overloading your knees and you reduce your chances of developing knee problems and a strained lower back. Pushing hard gears adds additional strain to your lower back. Furthermore, it was reported in the June 1992 issue of *Runner's World* that a high cadence has a cross-over effect on running! The faster you spin on the bike, the more your legs become conditioned to pumping faster and the more speed you will have when running. For example, cycling at 60 r.p.m. is the same as running an 8:30 minute mile; cycling at 90 r.p.m. is the same as running a 6:45 mile, and cycling at 100 r.p.m. is the same as running a 5:45 mile. Improvement in high-cadence cycling, therefore, will have cross-over benefits in running . . . and that's smart training!

In addition, research shows that by riding in a slightly advanced seating position (this usually means setting your seat at a steeper angle which will cause you to feel like you are pushing backwards with your legs; it also tends to feel more aggressive than the conventional riding position) your upper body tends to stay more relaxed and you tax your running muscles less. This technique may help you to conserve more energy thereby allowing you to run better after cycling. If you want to try this, seek out a good bike shop and experiment with gradual seat adjustments. As you use a more advanced seat position, you may have to adjust your handle bar stem as well.

3. As one study reported several years ago, if you can travel at 18 m.p.h. on a flat grade your speed will slow to about 6 m.p.h. when climbing a six percent grade. So learning to climb hills efficiently is important. When on an ascent, try to stay in the saddle as long as you can. This improves aerodynamics, power transfer and allows a smoother cadence. When necessary, you can climb out of the saddle for the tough parts or for a burst of speed. Remember to pace yourself so that you can "crest" the hill, that is, as you reach the top, you should be able to maintain your speed and shortly thereafter begin to accelerate again. If you despise hill climbing, consider getting into the gym and developing leg power so that hills can become fun or else move to the prairies and pray for wind-free days.

4. If you are not pedaling on the descent, clamp your knees to the top tube for stability and decreased wind resistance. Try to maintain your tuck for speed and on those fast corners, point the inside knee out for direction and stability. While some riders will bring their hands in close to the stem, it is advisable to keep your hands near the brake hoods just in case a pothole suddenly appears.

5. Practice your aerodynamic position in training so that your lower back can adapt to the stress. Keep switching your riding position so that your back doesn't cramp and so that your hands and neck will also not become sore or numb.

6. Strength training is a very effective way of improving your overall riding strength. Most accomplished cyclists prefer to focus on their weight training program during the off-season (fall and winter). Some of the basic exercises you might consider incorporating into your program are included in this chapter and in Chapter 8.

7. While flexibility may not make you go faster, it will improve your overall range of motion thereby reducing the risk of stress-related injuries. Stretching, therefore, should be part of your regular program.

8. For those of us living in cooler climates, training in cool, or even cold, weather is par for the course. In Alberta we often have beautiful sunny winter days that are extremely cold. It is important in these cases to guard against windchill which can lead to frostbite. In addition to wearing quality products made from moisture-transporting, synthetic materials like polypropylene, there are a number of other practical ways to make your ride more enjoyable:

   ▸ Start your ride by heading into the wind so that you don't have to freeze on the return after working up a sweat.

   ▸ Don't wear heavy clothes. Wear several light layers instead.

   ▸ If you want to drink, take a hot beverage in your water bottle (it won't freeze as fast as a cold drink).

   ▸ Wear light clothing that is readily visible. Motorists are not used to sharing the road with cyclists in the winter.

   ▸ Carry extra tires and inner tubes as you are likely to encounter more road debris than usual.

▸ Don't stop for long breaks after you've warmed up as you will find the windchill more uncomfortable.

▸ Don't ride more than ninety minutes in subfreezing conditions.

▸ Given the risk of windchill and road debris, consider using a mountain bike as an alternative to a road bike. A mountain bike will slow you down because of its less aerodynamic design thereby reducing wind resistance.

SAFETY

A few final points that should be self-evident, but given the statistics for bicycle-related accidents, we will reiterate them – for safety's sake!

▸ Always ride with caution.

▸ Obey all traffic rules.

▸ Avoid riding side by side unless you are on a designated cycling path.

▸ Never go anywhere without your helmet securely fastened.

Now you should have more than enough material to make an informed consumer choice, and to refine your current skills. We are now ready to take the next step forward – running.

Chapter 7

Running

Of the three sports involved in the triathlon, running is the most familiar and comfortable for newcomers. Unlike swimming or cycling, running is a weight-bearing exercise in which your legs absorb the pounding of your body while in the other sports you have either water or a bike to support you. Running, therefore, is the hardest on your body, and in this chapter we will discuss ways of improving your technique and speed while reducing the risk of injury. First, though, let's look at the bewildering array of equipment available in order to determine which is best for you.

· As your legs become accustomed to pumping faster when running, you will find that your cycling cadence will improve also.

· Visualization and relaxation may not appear to directly help your running, but if you keep track of your emotions and performances, you will notice the difference these techniques make.

· The more relaxed you are when you run, the faster you will go.

RUNNING ATTIRE

As any runner knows, running generates a considerable amount of body heat. Unlike cycling, where you can enjoy the cooling effect of moving at high speeds, it is quite a challenge to stay cool while running. The following is a list of apparel that you should consider if you wish to improve your comfort while running.

▶ *Running Socks.* Unlike street or cycling socks, running socks are cushioned to protect your feet from blisters and they are designed to keep your feet dry. These highly practical socks also keep your shoes from smelling!

▶ *Hats.* You lose a considerable amount of heat through the top of your head – especially in winter. It is a good idea, then, to wear hats, especially in cold weather. In summer, wearing a light hat can protect you from sunburn and heat exhaustion.

▶ *Sunglasses.* Aside from cutting the glare of the sun, sunglasses serve a practical role in UV protection. Numerous support straps are available to help keep your glasses in place while you run.

▶ *Gloves.* You may have seen races where the runners were scantily clad yet wore light gloves. These gloves are worn to prevent heat loss through the hands. This is an ideal way to maintain warmth without being encumbered by heavy clothing.

▶ *Running Tights.* You may recall the days of running in sweats and boldly patterned tights. Today, anything is acceptable so long as you can move freely. The best tights wick away any perspiration leaving your skin feeling dry. The same is true for upper body clothing. In winter, lightweight thermal polypropylene clothing is recommended. Its wicking properties will keep your skin dry and comfortable when the weather is chilly.

▶ *Shoes.* Running shoes are like people. They come in many shapes, sizes, colors, levels of stability, and even temperament. Like a good partner, a well-fitting shoe is not always easy to find. Furthermore, the most common or popular or expensive brand may not be the type for you.

Do not let a store clerk sell you any shoe unless the recommendation is based on the criteria listed in this chapter. Buying a pair of running shoes can be a major financial investment, so take the time to find a shoe that suits all of your needs. Many of the better shops will let you take shoes for a test run around the block or they may even have a treadmill in the store.

Well-trained staff can tell you which particular type of shoe you need, but a little observation of your own can determine this just as well. For example, look at a pair of your well-used running shoes. Does the sole tend to wear down in a particular manner? Consider the kind of mileage you run and on what type of surfaces you train (e.g., soft pathways, concrete or trails). If your shoes show excessive wear on the insides of the soles, that is, if the arch is flattened or the heel is tilted over, then you have a pronation problem. This means that your foot rolls from the outside to the inside. Shoes with excessive wear on the outside of the sole indicate a supination problem. Either condition results in sore tendons on the affected side. Perhaps you may be a heel striker (in which case your shoes will show signs of excessive heel wear), or a toe runner, or maybe you suffer from "floppy" feet where your feet roll from side to side as opposed to "rigid" feet (in which the heel-to-toe push-off is strong and stable).

These problems can be corrected to a certain extent by purchasing the right type of shoes. If you have serious foot problems, you should consider seeing a podiatrist, a chiropractor, or some other health care practitioner who can address the cause of the problem as opposed to simply treating the symptom. And since we all have biomechanical idiosyncrasies, it isn't just a matter of buying the best-looking shoe, or the pair that is the least expensive.

Once you have had your running style analyzed and a shoe recommended, then ask to take a trial run before putting your money down. (I have changed running shoe brands numerous times over the years. Although different companies have offered different incentives, I have always run with the shoes that seem to best suit my running style.)

In terms of shoe sizing, you should have about one-half inch or a thumb digit's worth of room between your big toe and the front of the shoe's toe box.

Another thing you need to decide is whether you need a 'slip lasted' or a 'board lasted' shoe. A 'last' is a molded form that gives the shoe its shape and structure. In a slip lasted shoe the midsole and and upper are sewn together, while a board lasted shoe will glue these two parts together. A knowledgeable store clerk will explain to you the type of last and the type of shoe you need. If you prefer a shoe which offers extra support and less flexibility, then look for a board-lasted shoe, one in which a piece of fiberboard is placed between the heel and mid-foot. On the other hand, if you prefer a more flexible shoe and do not require as much stability, then get a slip-lasted shoe. In slip last construction, the sole and midsole materials are usually glued directly to the cloth upper. Shoe shape is also variable. Look at your feet or step on a cement floor with wet feet to determine whether you need a straight or curved shoe. Get the shoe that mirrors the shape of your foot.

Consider buying two pairs of shoes for training and alternate their use. You will get longer wear out of them, and if one needs mending or gets soaked, you will have a back-up pair. Once you know which brand you prefer then you can look for sales.

You should buy training shoes that complement your weight. Men over 160 pounds should wear a heavier shoe while men 140–160 pounds can wear a light to medium weight trainer. Men under 140 pounds can go with lightweight trainers or even consider a woman's shoe – assuming you can find the right size. Conversely, women 140 pounds and over should consider wearing a man's shoe. Women under 140 pounds should select from the women's models – keeping in mind the criteria mentioned in this chapter.

In time, you may find that your shoes are no longer satisfactory. For example, your running style or your feet may have changed. New runners often notice their feet flatten out after several months of regular running. Take advantage of innovations in shoe design in order to obtain greater comfort, speed, shock absorption and most of all to keep pace with the changing needs of your feet.

Before we look at what is inside a running shoe, we need to talk about the racing flat. If you have ever watched marathons or 10 km runs you are likely to see the elite runners wearing very light running shoes. These are referred to as racing flats. In order to be light, however, these shoes must give up some durability, support and general comfort – all in the name of saving a few ounces. Given that most runners and triathletes will not be able to optimize the advantages of lighter shoes over a 10 km distance, you are better off using your training shoes or lightweight trainers. The added degree of support and comfort might make the difference between running one race or running several throughout the season.

If you are running in a marathon or Ironman race the advantages of wearing lighter shoes will be apparent over 26.2 miles (42 km). But you will need to do some long runs in your flats to be sure you can go the distance without too much discomfort. From a financial standpoint, good racing flats may not offer the best return on your investment, especially when you take into consideration their short lifespan.

INSIDE THE SHOE – USING INSERTS

If you are at all serious about running, you should consider buying separate inserts. There are many on the market. They range from the standard polypropylene footbeds which appear in most running shoes, to the high-tech custom graphite inserts which offer greater support and durability. For more serious foot problems, sports clinics often have qualified people who can make specialized orthotics.

Some of the newer orthotics can be easily reheated and remolded to adjust to changes in your feet. Also, if the initial configuration is for some reason uncomfortable you can simply redo the inserts. These highly practical inserts are available from a variety of health practitioners such as chiropractors, naturopaths and orthopedists.

When buying shoes, then, be sure the existing inserts can be removed. This is not possible with all racing flats, although, most running shoe companies no longer glue insoles into their quality shoes. Inserts that come in running shoes are often of poor quality and are not recommended if you want to get the most out of your shoe. An additional benefit of some orthotic inserts is that you can transfer them to other shoes, even dress shoes, depending on the type of shoe and type of fit.

WHEN TO REPLACE THOSE BELOVED SHOES?

Over the years I have become quite attached to certain shoes. They fit well, suited my running style perfectly and I felt like I could run in them for the rest of my life. Whenever I ran in a new pair, however, I could instantly feel the improvement in support and comfort and yet I would keep the old pair for a nostalgic fun run. We do not recommend you acquire this bad habit. I just want to illustrate how attached you can get to something that has given you so much satisfaction but has outworn its useful life.

The following list summarizes the average lifespan of sports and fitness shoes, assuming that you exercise regularly (approximately three or more times per week). It should be noted, however, that individual traits such as weight, technique and even the running terrain will affect the lifespan of your shoe. If you keep a training log, note when you bought the shoes. Do not rely on your memory and injuries to tell you it is time to check and replace your shoes.

SHOE TYPE	HOW LONG THEY LAST WITH REGULAR USE
Aerobic	6–12 months
Cycling	1–2 years
Cross-training	9–12 months
Running	500–600 miles/3–6 months
Racing flats	1 season of racing (7–10 races)

RUNNING TECHNIQUE

Contrary to what some people would believe, there is no perfect running form. It is critical that you be aware of your own unique and natural style if you are to achieve optimum performance. If running feels like a struggle then you are not working in harmony with your natural style. Comfort and ease of movement should be your objective. There are, however, a number of fundamental principles you can work on to improve your form and, ultimately, your speed:

▸ Keep your upper body (head, neck and shoulders) relatively erect. Think tall. This way you are not fighting gravity and it is easier to relax.

▸ Your face and shoulders should be relaxed. Be aware of them as you run. Your facial muscles should feel as if they are bouncing. By learning the art of upper-body relaxation, you can even reduce tension in your shoulders, neck and face.

▸ Your arm swing should be natural and not exaggerated. Your arms should be slightly bent and move in a relatively straight forward and backward motion. All body motions should be directed to propelling you forward. Look at pictures of Carl Lewis, perhaps one of the finest form runners in recent history – even his fingers are pointed forward as he pumps his arms back and forth like pistons.

▸ Your hands should be relaxed but not limp and your thumb and pointer finger should touch lightly. As you run, imagine your hands leading you forward.

- Be sure not to rotate your upper body – especially your shoulders. People with tight shoulders have a tendency to do this. Many neophyte runners show tension and stress in their shoulders when running. Excess upper body rotation just means that you will have to expend more effort and probably make more frequent visits to your favorite chiropractor.

- For runs of 10 km or longer, you must minimize knee lift. Lift your knees only high enough so that you can get proper leg extension without overstriding or understriding. Your knee lift and forward movement should feel natural. As you plant your foot, your heel should come down naturally without excessive force.

- Practice form from time to time! Ken Souza, once one of the world's top duathletes, recommends skipping drills as a way to teach your body to stay erect and to develop proper foot plant and stride. A standard drill begins with five sets of twenty to thirty meters of skipping. Then do another five sets of thirty to fifty meters at an easy jogging pace. Do more sets to focus on keeping tall, relaxing your arms, shoulders and upper torso, and then do a final set focusing only on staying relaxed. Believe it or not, the more relaxed you are when you run, the faster you will go.

- As you follow through with your stride, you should be pushing off lightly with your toes, and your heel should kick up close to your gluts before it comes forward again. To see this technique in action, watch sprinters when they run. They kick up in an exaggerated way, but they get tremendous forward power from their follow-through. Be light and quick on your feet. Some runners prefer a type of shuffle style with minimal knee and heel kick but it is not the norm. Though it is economical for ultra triathlon or Ironman distance races, the top runners seldom do this. Refer to Figure 7.1 to see what a proper running form should look like.

▸ Since breathing is necessary to transport oxygen through the body, breathe normally and rhythmically. A good breathing pattern can also relax and integrate your body and mind. Some runners maintain a steady rhythm by breathing in through their nose and out through their mouth. In cold weather this breathing method warms the air more than breathing in through the mouth thereby allowing you to run with greater comfort.

▸ Runners are more injury prone than cyclists or swimmers because they often run more than their body can handle, neglect to do proper warm-ups or cool-downs, or do too many intervals. Running puts tremendous stress on the body therefore you should pay close attention to how your running is affecting you and adapt your training accordingly.

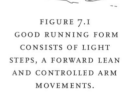

FIGURE 7.1
GOOD RUNNING FORM CONSISTS OF LIGHT STEPS, A FORWARD LEAN AND CONTROLLED ARM MOVEMENTS.

▸ Finally, Jeff Galloway, a former American Olympic-distance runner, offers three useful form tips denoted by the acronym CHP.

Chest up

Hips forward

Push off strongly with your foot

He suggests practicing these form tips at an easy pace until they become comfortable.

RUNNING WARM-UPS AND COOL-DOWNS

Warm-up properly before any physical activity. If it is cold outside or if you're stiff, you should walk for a few minutes. Then, when you feel comfortable, jog at an easy pace for about ten minutes before you reach your training pace. (If you are warming up for a race then jog easily for ten to fifteen minutes.) Follow with some light stretching and then some accelerations (e.g., five to eight repeats of 75 to 100 meters). Take plenty of rest between each acceleration. Then conclude your warm-up with an easy three to five minute jog.

For your cool-down, jog easily for about 1.5 miles (about two km). If you are really tired, alternate jogging with a moderately paced walk. Your muscles will thank you for it.

SMART RUNNING — IN THE POOL

A number of successful runners and triathletes have incorporated pool running into their programs to minimize the stress on the body during training. Olympic medalist Lynn Williams, once Canada's top 3,000 meter specialist, gave a lot of the credit to her success to her pool workouts. Joan Samuelson, another Olympic medalist, used pool running as part of her 1984 Olympic marathon program. Donna Peters, a very successful duathlete, used pool running to help her recover from a serious cycling accident in 1990. Donna then finished a very strong fourth at the 1992 Triathlon World Championship in Muskoka, Ontario.

If you do take to the pool, use a flotation device that will enable you to move freely while still keeping you afloat. When running in the pool, try to simulate running on land. That is, concentrate on your form, staying erect, using your arms and getting good knee lift. For added resistance you can use your hands like paddles. A good pool workout can be done in thirty to forty-five minutes. After a five to ten minute warm-up, start doing one to two minute sprints. Your heart rate will not be as high as on land, and, without the weight-bearing stress of land running, you can tolerate more intervals. As it is easy to overdo it when you are in the water, you should pay attention to your body and muscles to avoid fatigue and overstraining.

MENTAL PREPARATION

Many of us run but never reach our potential. In his book *The Total Runner*, sports psychologist Jerry Lynch suggests we don't reach our potential because most of us don't know how to. Mental preparation in any sport is as important as the physical preparation, although many athletes neglect this part of their training. Learn to visualize, practice relaxation techniques and get a massage once in a while. These may not appear to directly help your running, but if you keep track of your emotions and your performances, you will begin to see changes if you incorporate these activities into your lifestyle and training program.

RUNNING DRILLS

Running drills are intended to strengthen the key running muscles, improve rhythm, comfort and form and enable you to run faster. I have summarized some excellent drills you can practice and incorporate into your training. For more detail and information, you might like to get Jeff Galloway's book on running – a classic in its field. Otherwise, sign up for an instructional clinic and don't be afraid to ask a high school, college or university track and field coach any questions about your training.

Earlier we recommended using a skipping drill to improve your form. Other drills which can be incorporated into your program are included below. Remember, always do a proper warm-up and cool-down – a two to three mile jog before and a one mile jog after. Build intensity. Do not make any drastic changes. Listen to your body and monitor your heart rate. Let these indicators dictate the rate of change in your training. If you are a multisport athlete only do the drills once a week. If running is your only serious sport, do the drills twice per week.

► Uphill repeats build the strength needed for speed. The famous running coach Arthur Lydiard (who some claim to have invented jogging with his long slow run workouts) maintains that hills are the only beneficial type of resistance training for runners and that hill workouts will improve your overall running skills. Using a hill with a ten to fifteen percent grade, you should gradually build distance and number of repeats from 100 to 800 meters. Begin with three to four repeats and build when you feel strong enough to maintain the form and rhythm you established on the flats.

► Because of the demand placed on your body by hill running, incorporate only one of these sessions per week. As this is a strength-building drill, it is best done in the off-season. Experiment slowly and carefully and adapt it wherever necessary to fit into your own training program.

► Running downhill can improve leg turnover speed and teach you to lengthen your stride as far as possible while maintaining comfort. You can use the same hill for uphill and downhill drills. As you go down, lean forward slightly and focus on staying in control, running smoothly and staying relaxed. If you find yourself slapping your feet down or striking excessively with your heel, you are overstriding and should adjust your stride until you are running smoothly.

► The rapid high knee-lifts are good for the hip flexors, gluts and developing lower leg strength. This exercise involves leaning slightly forward and taking short quick strides in which you lift your knees to waist level. Galloway suggests that for this drill you pretend you are walking on ice. This is *not* a speed drill. You should focus on form and flexibility.

The kick-out drill improves the flexibility of your ankles. Use the same format as with the knee-lifts but this time bring your striding foot up to your butt and then reach out as if you were doing the goose step. The kick-out foot should reach about forty-five degrees. This drill can be done a little faster than the knee-lift.

▸ If you really want a good workout in which you use all the major leg muscles then combine knee lifts and kick-outs on a hill with a grade of around ten percent. The distance covered per repeat need only be between 30–75 meters.

Bart Yasso, Race and Event Director with *Runner's World* magazine, has devised the simplest marathon training program with which you can predict your finishing time. Starting several months before the big event, time yourself over an 800-meter run. Be realistic about how hard you can go, then slowly build up the number of repeats each week until you are doing ten per week at the same pace. Each repeat should be followed by one 400-meter recovery run. The duration of a single repeat will translate into the hours and minutes it will take to run the marathon. For example, a time of 2:50 per repeat will equal a 2 hour and 50 minute marathon time, while a time of 3:08 per repeat will mean that you will run a marathon in 3 hours and 8 minutes. Of course, you will still need to do your basic mileage to condition your body to meet the demands of a marathon.

YOU AND THE ELEMENTS

Running produces a considerable amount of body heat. This is why many runners prefer running in cooler weather but riding or swimming in warmer conditions. Here are some basic pointers for cold-weather running.

- Heat is dissipated mainly through your head and hands. If it is cold, you should wear a hat and light gloves. Men should provide extra protection to their vital parts as nylon offers no defense against penile frostbite – something you don't want to experience – trust me, I know! Either wear several layers of clothes, a jockstrap, tight-fitting wool underwear, or the special winter underwear that can readily be found in cross-country ski stores.

- Breathing cold air can be uncomfortable. But it is almost impossible to freeze your lungs. If you must run in the extreme cold, wrap a scarf around your mouth or get a neoprene face mask. These masks are great, for not only do they protect your lungs, but most have a nose guard and covers for your lower ear lobes. I have used them to run comfortably in temperatures of $-22°F$ ($-30°C$) and colder.

- If you do need to bundle up, use light, layered clothing. Polypropylene or wool (if your skin is not too sensitive) work well.

- If the conditions are cold and wet, there is nothing better than a waterproof breathable shell jacket. It will keep you dry by wicking the sweat away from your body.

- Finally, a word of common sense: always start your run in the direction of the wind or rain so your body can heat up before you turn back and face the elements.

Now, if the weather is hot you have other things to consider:

- The most important danger of hot weather running is fluid loss. Running creates a lot of body heat that is kept in check by sweating, which can dehydrate you faster than you think. You can dress lightly to keep your body cool, but you will still perspire. Your best defense is to drink regularly throughout the day and frequently during your runs – especially in those runs lasting more than an hour. Most races have water aid stations every mile and, depending on your tolerance to the heat, you should consider taking water at each station. *Do not let your thirst guide your fluid intake.* If you do you will dehydrate quickly!

- Today, most good running attire is designed to wick away perspiration and to offer the coolest run possible. Contrary to some beliefs, when running in the heat, it is better to wear something light than nothing at all as apparel shields the sun. This is why you often see runners wearing a light sun cap or visor. Finally, in order to avoid chafing in the heat, wear loose clothing.

- When you are running, heat can be a "killer." This is because your body loses a lot of water in an effort to stay cool, thus draining it of vital energy. Therefore, if you plan on racing in the heat, train in the heat. This acclimatization training must include drinking more water than usual in order to keep your fluid levels stable. During my prime racing years I used to intentionally train in weather that simulated race conditions. I swam in cold lakes rather than pools and rode and ran in the heat of the day. I became so accustomed to the heat that I looked forward to racing in the heat – it became an ally rather than a foe.

  If you train in cool weather, simply wear extra clothing to simulate hot conditions. Many Canadians who race in the Hawaii Ironman in October have difficulty with the heat because our warm summer days have long since given way to the cool conditions of autumn. Therefore, if you cannot afford the extra two weeks to fly over and adjust to the heat – improvise!

  Finally, whenever training in the heat, err on the side of drinking *too much* water and increase your mileage and intensity *gradually*.

RUNNING INJURIES

You are more likely to incur a running injury before you suffer an injury from swimming or cycling. One recent survey found that over seventy percent of all runners have suffered at least one major injury as a result of their training, with the knee suffering more injuries than any other body part.

According to running guru Jeff Galloway, the causes of knee injuries include: worn-out shoes, running too much, sudden increases in distance and inadequate shoe cushioning. Injuries can also result from biomechanical foot problems such as rigid feet or floppy feet. Therefore, you need to pay close attention to what you wear on your feet and how you train.

A common ailment afflicting many dedicated athletes is not knowing when to stop. For example, have you ever found yourself trying to "run out" a pain or taking some other measure which enables you to keep running in spite of physical discomfort? If this is the case, you need a reality check! It is likely you are overtraining or even addicted to your training regime. Always listen to your body; it will tell you when you have had enough.

Another easy way to incur injuries is to be the "weekend warrior." This is someone who has too little time to work out during the week, and overcompensates by packing too much in on the weekend. The weekend warrior will sooner burn out than enjoy the benefits of a balanced, holistic lifestyle. If you are one of these people, you should review the principles of time management set out in Chapter 2.

If you are lucky and an injury goes away of its own accord – great! If it persists, however, your body will begin to adjust and compensate over time and the unfortunate thing is that you may not even realize it. Any compensation places tremendous strain on the musculoskeletal system and so it may not only aggravate the existing problem but will likely create additional ones!

Unfortunately, the body's pain mechanism is not a very good barometer for telling us when an injury is forthcoming. Painful symptoms usually only occur after the injury has manifested itself. By training smart, keeping your mileage to a manageable level and paying attention to your body's signals, you reduce your risk of injury. Here are some basic guidelines to help you distinguish between an injury and a temporary ache. An injury is characterized by the following signs:

- *Compensation.* The ailment prevents you from running in your natural form.

- *Persistence.* The ailment lasts for more than a week.

- *Escalation.* The problem gets worse.

- *Swelling.* A simple comparison of each of your feet, ankles or knees will indicate that something is wrong.

- *Pain.* If you have reached this stage, it may be time to seek help. You can mask the pain with medication, but remember, this does not address the problem!

Now that we have examined the sports of triathlon, let's see how weight training can give you the strength and endurance to carry you through these events.

Chapter 8

Weight Training for Strength and Endurance

As you probably noticed, the title of this chapter does not say anything about bodybuilding. For our purposes, the aim of weight training is to increase your strength to weight ratio and your endurance. Good rock climbers tend to be lean in build yet very strong. The ability to pull your body upward with one arm, and in some cases a few fingers, requires considerable strength. High jumpers must have good leg strength in order to jump to impressive heights and gymnasts must be strong in order to complete all their routines. These, and many other sports, require varying degrees of strength in situations where weight could be a disadvantage. Duathlons and triathlons also fall within this general classification.

At the 1992 World Triathlon Championship in Muskoka, Ontario I watched some of the lead racers drop to the back of the pack as the race wore on because physically, they could not stand up to the demanding undulating course. Three competitors in particular who were just coming off successful Ironman and other long distance races were too drained to maintain their pace even though they had held their own in the swim and bike portions.

- The aim of weight training is to increase your strength to weight ratio and your endurance.

- Weight training is a very effective way of improving your overall cycling strength.

- Weight training improves your body posture and mechanics.

The running course required considerable strength in order to power over the bigger hills and to run across a soggy grass field.

The benefits of weight training should not be overlooked by anyone interested in staying active – especially anyone serious about participating competitively. Do I hear you say you already have enough things to do? Do triathletes really need to build up extra strength and endurance? These are good questions. Consider the following:

► Swimming involves moving through water which is almost twelve times more dense than air – now that's resistance training.

► Cycling requires leg power to propel the bike along the flats and up hills, and strong stomach muscles are required to support your back in the aero position.

► Running is a high-impact activity that can create a great deal of stress on your limbs. One recent article estimated that a 150-pound runner produces 450 pounds of force per step! And given that a short course triathlon is 10 km, that works out to about 6,200 steps or 1,395 tons of force being transmitted through your legs and up into your body. If you can't quite imagine this, try bench pressing any weight until you have amassed the equivalent of 1,395 tons of weight lifted!

Few triathlon or duathlon books have any discussion about weight training, but, it is not foreign to the sport. In fact, Mark Allen recently attributed some of his longevity in the triathlon to weight training and, judging by the physical appearance of some of the competitors at the swim start line, many others do so as well.

According to bodybuilding guru Bill Pearl, athletes in most sports can benefit from weight training. The American College of Sports Medicine (ACSM) recommends at least two weekly sessions of resistance training and suggests that during each session you work both the major upper and lower muscle groups.

ADVANTAGES OF WEIGHT TRAINING

- additional strength for power surges and acceleration
- muscular endurance for sustained effort
- muscle groups become balanced which reduces the risk of injury and facilitates recovery from injury
- enhanced general body proportion
- improved body posture and body mechanics
- aerobic benefit from weight training sessions lasting twelve minutes or more
- improved flexibility as muscles, tendons and ligaments are strengthened
- significant scientific evidence shows that weight training helps prevent diseases such as osteoporosis

Weight training conditions the muscles to exert more force. Repeated efforts over a period of time increase the amount of actin and myosin in the muscle fibers which translates into greater strength. Muscular endurance can also be improved through proper weight training. There is, however, a trade-off. If you concentrate on strength training alone (heavy weights and few repetitions), then you sacrifice endurance (which can be improved by low to moderate weights and many repetitions). The bottom line is that strong muscles won't fatigue as easily as weak muscles and this improves endurance.

THE IMPORTANCE OF WEIGHT TRAINING

Triathlons and duathlons are primarily aerobic activities. At certain times, however, you might want to call upon your anaerobic reservoir to accelerate in the swim, overtake another racer, sprint up a hill, or even just break away from the pack. To do this the muscle groups are activated in a certain order. Aerobic activity depends on slow-twitch muscle fibers while more contractile force requires intermediate fibers. Sooner or later these fibers become exhausted and the body resorts to the fast-twitch (white) fibers. The result is anaerobic exertion. If these muscle fibers are untrained, you will not have explosive power and will run out of steam quickly. The only way to build this vital energy reserve is through focused training which should involve specific weight training exercises.

Each of the three triathlon sports use different muscles and everyone has some muscles which are stronger than others. Therefore, you should concentrate on those exercises which best address your weaknesses. Consider the run, which is usually the most taxing of the three triathlon events. It is not only the last event in a triathlon but it is more physically demanding than swimming or cycling. A runner's physical weakness will reveal itself in a slackened pace and an awkward gait. If, for example, your hamstrings or quadriceps begin to fatigue, your legs will tighten up and your stride will shorten; or as your shoulders weaken from trying to keep yourself moving forward, your arms and neck muscles will tighten and you will lose the ability to pump strongly up the hills or surge to the finish line. Regardless of how well you may have swum or cycled, if you begin to lose power on the run, it could mean the difference between a great performance and surviving the race.

FREE WEIGHTS OR MACHINES?

If you ask any serious bodybuilder or athlete whether it is better to train with free weights or machines, they will most likely argue that free weights are the foundation of any good training program. Free weights allow you to work specific muscles and improve body proportion, balance, coordination and symmetry. For example, try the bench press on a machine and then try free weights – you will notice a difference!

Having said this, machines allow for fairly rapid movement from one exercise to the next. They tend to be safer and you can change weights more quickly. In addition, they are more fun and inviting than those gray free weights. Machines also require little supervision. If you use free weights consider having a spotter who can help you in the event that the weight suddenly becomes to much to bear. A partner can also make the workout more enjoyable. After all, isn't it more fun to share something good?

THE PARTIALS PARADOX

Since many of us do not have unlimited time to train, we either compromise our weight training workouts or do not do them at all. If you would like to include weight training as part of your fitness program, then "partials" might be one alternative to spending long hours in the gym.

Fitness consultants John Little and Peter Sisco suggest that it is possible to increase muscle power by not only doing *fewer* weight sessions but by moving through only *part* of the potential range of motion in a given exercise. The technique is called "Power Factor Training." They argue that in order to gain muscle size and strength you only need to move a weight through the range of motion in which you are strongest. This usually involves only two to four inches (5–10 cm) of travel. By overloading your strongest muscles you also recruit and stimulate all the complementary ones.

Secondly, they point out that we need far more time to recover from an intense workout than we realize. They found that strength training three or more times per week can be counterproductive! According to their approach, once or twice a week is all that is needed to produce gains. Although I have experimented with this approach and find a lot of merit in it, I suggest a more conventional routine of about three workouts per week. This program works particularly well in the off-season as long as regular workouts are kept up.

Little and Sisco's total body workout program can involve as few as nine exercises. The exercises include: lat pull-downs, dead lifts, bench press, leg press, toe press, shoulder press, shrugs, preacher curls and dips. They consider abdominals as part of your aerobic training and they recommend 4 to 6 sets of each exercise, 10 to 30 reps per set, increasing the weight each set.

WHEN SHOULD I WEIGHT TRAIN?

Since there is no set protocol for when to do your weight sessions, we suggest you experiment in consultation with a personal trainer or athletic coach. Some days I lift weights after my sport-specific workouts so that I can get better results from my workout. On other days, when I want to work on endurance and strength building, I will do the weight sessions before my workout – e.g., a leg session in the morning followed by a bike ride. The legs have already been taxed and it becomes essential to ride efficiently and effectively in order to complete the session.

If you do a strength or endurance session before a sport-specific activity, do not make it a high-intensity workout, as you will increase the risk of injury and place undue stress on your body.

HOW TO GET THE MOST OUT OF YOUR WEIGHT TRAINING PROGRAM

Safety

Since you are working with weights, safety should always be a concern. Sloppy form such as quick thrusts or jerks can result in sudden injury. Use a smooth and steady motion – one which nearly approximates the speed that you would use the muscle group during the swim, bike or run. Don't try to lift weights that are well beyond your comfort zone. While it may seem impressive, lifting too heavy a weight increases your chances of injury. In this respect it is very much like overtraining.

Inhale when lifting weights, exhale when lowering. Unless you are already well versed in weight training, consult a fitness instructor at your local club or community center before starting. For the CDN$30–$50 they might charge, a few lessons on "how to" will make it a more enjoyable activity and reduce your risk of hurting yourself.

Flexibility

Remember that each sport has different flexibility requirements. You need sufficient flexibility to go through the range of motion required for the sport otherwise you will be hampered by a lack of movement. For triathletes, improving flexibility should be part of your training program. Believe it or not, strength and endurance training, if done properly, will improve your range of motion. You won't and don't need to look like the Incredible Hulk in order to be strong. You should, however, include regular stretching exercises and yoga in your flexibility program.

Warming Up

All weight sessions should be preceded by a ten to fifteen minute warm-up. Do a yoga sun salutation (described below), ride a stationary bike, work out on the cross-country machine, use a Stairmaster®, or do anything that will allow you to elevate your heart rate, warm up your muscles and work up a light sweat.

Dr. Kenneth Cooper, founder of the Institute for Aerobic Research in Dallas, Texas, found that jumping rope was one of the most effective ways to burn calories and improve cardiovascular health. Ten minutes of jumping rope will burn as many calories as thirty minutes of either jogging, swimming or cycling. A 165-pound man can burn up to 850 calories during an hour of jumping rope. The only other activity which might rival jumping rope is cross-country skiing (you can use an indoor ski machine as well). Consider incorporating either or both of these activities into your warm-up routine.

SUN SALUTATION "GET UP AND GO"

This set of dynamic stretches, which is based on the sun cycle used in many yoga routines, is one of the most comprehensive you can incorporate into your daily routine. Unless you are injured, pregnant or menstruating, the sun salutation offers a safe set of stretches to do. Doing the full cycle helps to deepen breathing. The cycle also boosts circulation and helps to energize the whole body. The routine should be done slowly with attention given to proper breathing and stretching.

1. Start in a standing position with body and mind in a calm and focused state. Take a few deep breaths to focus your attention. (Figure 8.1 – Move 1)

2. With feet together, stretch your arms upward, keeping them shoulder width apart. As you do so, lift your rib cage and stretch your palms and fingers. Do not overextend your arms and make sure that your spine stays straight. Breathe in slowly as you execute the stretch. Remember to breathe deeply. (Move 2)

3. Bend from the hips and keep your back straight or slightly arched. Be sure to keep your feet flat on the floor, your legs straight and your head in line with your spine. Slowly exhale as you reach for the floor. Do not overstretch. This stretch is excellent for increasing the flexibility in hips, hamstrings and spine. (Move 3)

Figure 8.1 SUN SALUTATION

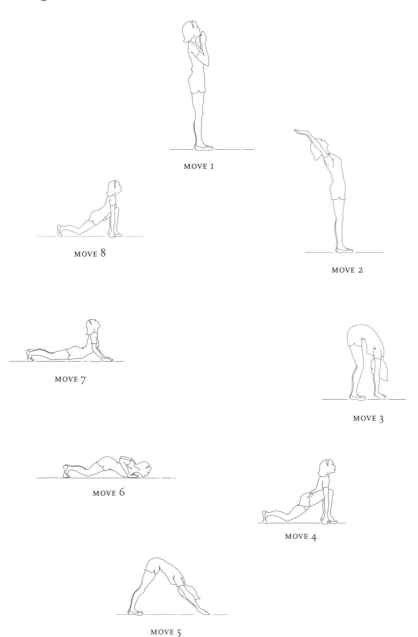

MOVE 1

MOVE 2

MOVE 3

MOVE 4

MOVE 5

MOVE 6

MOVE 7

MOVE 8

4. If at first you cannot reach the floor, bend your knees slightly until your palms lay flat on the floor. Support your weight on your hands then stretch your left leg behind you as you lift your torso up. Keep your bent knee ahead of your body. As you slide your leg back, breathe in slowly and lift your rib cage. Keep your head in line with your spine. (Move 4)

5. Bring your forward leg back and lift your hips up high. As you straighten out your legs, rise up on your toes. Let your spine stretch forward as your arms (still shoulder width apart) straighten at the same time. Your head should then drop between your shoulders. This motion should be done smoothly. Exhale throughout the stretch. If you feel comfortable, let your heels drop toward the floor. This is an excellent whole body stretch. (Move 5)

6. From this position, slowly lower your upper body so that your chin and head dip down toward the floor. Your body should be stretched and supported by your hands which are resting under your shoulders. If it is difficult to support your weight, you can rest your knees on the floor to help support your body weight. Breathe in throughout this movement. (Move 6)

7. From this horizontal position, gently lift your upper body. Your arms should be placed just in front of your shoulders. Keep your legs straight and your toes pointed. Lift from your upper back and arms. Tighten your buttock muscles and stretch your spine. Inhale throughout the lift. (Move 7)

8. Follow movement number 4, but this time move the right leg behind you. (Move 8)

9. Bring your body back up into the position described in point 5 and repeat moves 5–7.

   Complete the sun cycle by coming to a centered stance with your arms by your side. Focus on breathing deeply, relaxing your body and feeling energized.

You can repeat the same routines as many times as you like. Ideally it should be done for a minimum of five minutes or more until the body feels "alive."

You want to improve to a point where you can complete the sun cycle in a smooth and effortless fashion. Remember, do not strain yourself. If you find yourself having to strain, you should try doing only partial moves until your body is able to perform them properly.

Note: There are many variations of the sun salutation. This cycle includes most of the key movements but you might want to explore some of the other methods as you discover how energizing the exercise is.

HOW TO WORK OUT

To maximize the benefits of your program, work up to three (maximum four) weight sessions spaced evenly throughout the week. Each session should last forty-five to seventy-five minutes. Preferably begin your weight training session after your triathlon aerobic training. Although exceptions can be made, the main goal of weight training is to improve your triathlon/aerobic performance. Since you are not out to build muscle mass, you will want to treat your weight training as an aerobic activity. Therefore, try to keep moving between exercises so that in addition to strengthening your body, you are also building endurance. Do two or three exercises in succession so that you can move from one to the next without having to take long rests between sets – this is called a modified circuit training program. In this way you will feel comfortably tired at the end. If you wear a heart-rate monitor, you can check to see if you are in the heart-rate zone in which you will obtain aerobic benefit (i.e., sixty-five to eighty percent of your maximum heart rate).

Some athletes prefer to divide their upper- and lower-body workouts over separate days so that they do some weights each day they train. Upper-body workouts require less recovery time than lower body workouts. Since smaller muscle groups fatigue faster than the large ones, work on the larger muscle groups first. Research also indicates that if any part of your body should be treated differently, it is the *lumbar extensors* – primarily the muscles of the back. These muscles should be specifically exercised only once per week. A typical strength training sequence begins by working the abdominals then the thighs, chest, back, shoulders, triceps and biceps. Other athletes prefer to incorporate aerobic activity into their weight circuit to better simulate race conditions. For example, for half of your workout you might add a thirty to forty-five second aerobic exercise between each "station." You can cycle, run on the spot, jump rope or use the block (also known as the step). Not only does this give you variety, but as your muscle strength increases so will your stamina. Now that's smart training! Experiment with what works best for you – tailor your own program.

THE YEAR-ROUND TRAINING CYCLE

While in the past some athletes went into hibernation in the off-season, today it is generally recognized that good health and well-being require year-round attention. And just as we experience natural seasonal changes, so should you incorporate variation into your health and fitness program.

As noted in Chapter 4, you can design your training cycle to incorporate all the essential workouts by spreading them throughout the year at the times when they best suit your athletic needs. Weight training should be done during the off-season while endurance training is done in the pre-season and race season. Training during the race season should be less frequent so that you can concentrate on sport-specific activities.

Most experts suggest two to three workouts per week except during the peak racing phase when you can cut workouts altogether. Endurance athletes will want to use high reps with low to moderate weight (refer to the section on TRIMPs to calculate the ideal weight you should be lifting). As a triathlete, you should be interested in muscular endurance and strength, not bodybuilding *per se*. Remember to design your training program to fit your sports and your goals.

To look at the training cycle phases more closely, refer to Table 8.1 and Table 8.4.

Table 8.1 TRAINING CYCLE PHASES

	PREPARATORY		COMPETITIVE		RECOVERY
Training Phase	1	2	3	4	5
	Build Up Endurance	Maximum Strength	Conversion to Power	Maintain and/or Compete	Rest and Recover

PHASE 1: BUILD UP ENDURANCE

In the off-season, twenty to twenty-five percent of your total training volume should be strength and endurance training. This phase should last anywhere from two to six weeks.

▶ Develop an overall foundation of strength.

▶ Improve all muscle groups.

▶ Prepare muscles, tendons, joints and ligaments.

▶ Lift only a low to medium load, increasing the weight gradually to prevent accidents and injuries.

PHASE 2: MAXIMUM STRENGTH

Strength refers to the ability of muscles to produce force. It is measured by the amount of weight you can lift, press or pull in one movement, e.g., the maximum amount of weight you can bench press. During the maximum strength phase your focus will change.

This phase should last anywhere from one to three months (and will vary depending on your level of commitment). Here you will be developing power and endurance to go fast and long.

PHASE 3: CONVERSION TO POWER

The third phase of your periodization program is the conversion to power phase. This stage builds muscular endurance and should last anywhere from one to two months.

▸ If you are training for a triathlon you should focus on building strength for endurance.

▸ If you are training for a sprinting event, then focus on building strength for power.

▸ Use circuit workouts to meet your goals.

PHASE 4: MAINTAIN AND/OR COMPETE

The fourth phase requires a major reduction in intensity and volume. Here you maintain the strength and endurance you

---

MINI AND MACRO CYCLES

What happens if you want to race in January, March *and* October? This requires a little creative balance and experimentation. You will want to incorporate mini cycles, i.e., training cycles compressed into smaller segments of time. Macro cycles are based on the traditional notion of a race period covering a season (e.g., summer) and overlapping into another.

With the TRIMPS program developed by Dr. Banister (discussed in Chapter 12), it is possible to fine-tune your training cycle to accommodate a less-than-perfect triathlon/duathlon season. In other words, if you are going to race throughout the year or train over several seasons, you will likely want to create mini cycles. By using the TRIMPS program, you can structure the different phases so you do not lose any significant performance ability. Olympic athletes, for example, will have a series of mini, macro and super-macro cycles that will enable them to "be in the best shape ever" by the time they reach the Olympics.

have worked so hard to build. The duration of this phase will depend on how long your race season is and how much time you have between races.

- Balance your strength and endurance.
- Mix your workouts to reflect your needs. For example, shorter races require that you concentrate more on power while longer races require strength for endurance.
- Limit your workouts to two per week.

RECOVERY

Even the most dedicated athlete deserves a period of active and passive rest. This phase can last up to three weeks. The idea is to provide a mental and physical break from your routine. As noted earlier, any activity in this phase should be unstructured and geared toward having fun. If you must do weights, work at a low intensity with few repetitions.

SAMPLE STRENGTH/ENDURANCE PROGRAM

Table 8.2 offers a sample of the basic yet essential exercises that will work all the essential and primary support muscle groups required in triathlon. These exercises can be used as a general whole body training program regardless of the sport you pursue. Table 8.4 provides a suggested training cycle for a year-round program. You should not begin a weight training program without consulting a professional weight training consultant.

Table 8.2 WHOLE BODY WEIGHT TRAINING GUIDE

EXERCISES	SETS	REPS
WARM-UP/STRETCHING		
1. military grip bench press	3	12–15
2. straight-arm dumb-bell pullover ·	3	15
3. bicep curls	3	15
4. sit-ups (inclined bench—optional)	2–3	15–30
5. squats (machine or free)	3	15
* can alternate with leg press		
6. thigh extension on leg extension machine	3	25
7. leg curls (single or double leg)	3	25
8. hanging sit-ups	3	20–25
9. pullover	3	20
10. row (free or machine)	3	15
11. lateral and military press	3	20
Cool down/stretching		
OPTIONAL:		
12. shoulder press	3	15
13. dip for pectorals and triceps		
(if you are not strong enough,		
use a gravity machine if available)	3	6–12
14. lunges with free weights	3	10–12

If these exercises are done properly, with thirty to sixty second rests between each set, it will take you about an hour to complete. Try to do your weight training after any other workouts so they will not be affected by tired muscles. If you want to work on aerobic endurance and strength, however, then do weights beforehand.

Just as you would monitor your progress in your regular training program, keep track of your progress with the weights. Most clubs will provide you with a weight training chart to record your workouts. Otherwise, you could devise one similar to that shown below.

Table 8.3 STRENGTH TRAINING LOG

Date: From _____ to _____

EXERCISE	WEIGHTS/REPS/FREQUENCY	1 2 3 4 5 6 7 8 9 10
Squats		
Military Press		
Thigh Extension		
Etc.		

Table 8.4 ANNUAL STRENGTH TRAINING CYCLES

▶ JANUARY–FEBRUARY (Precompetitive)

EMPHASIS	INTENSITY	REPS	SETS	REST INTVLS	TIMES/WEEK
strength (2 wks)	80–95%	3–6	3–6	1–2 min	3
muscle endurance (2 wks)	65–80%	6–10	4–5	30–40 sec	3

▶ MARCH–APRIL (Precompetitive)

EMPHASIS	INTENSITY	REPS	SETS	REST INTVLS	TIMES/WEEK
strength (2 wks)	80–95%	3–6	4–6	1–2 min	3–4
power (2 wks)	85–100%	1–3	4–6	1–2 min	3–4

▶ APRIL–MAY (Transition)

EMPHASIS	INTENSITY	REPS	SETS	REST INTVLS	TIMES/WEEK
muscle endurance (3 wks)	65–80%	8–12	4–5	20–30 sec	2–3
power (1–2 wks)	85–100%	1–3	4–6	1–2 min	2–3

▶ JUNE–AUGUST (Competitive)

EMPHASIS	INTENSITY	REPS	SETS	REST INTVLS	TIMES/WEEK
muscle endurance	60–70%	12–30	2–3	20–30 sec	2

▶ SEPTEMBER–OCTOBER (Active Rest)

EMPHASIS	INTENSITY	REPS	SETS	REST INTVLS	TIMES/WEEK
muscle endurance	60%	12–30	2	30–40 sec*	1–2

▶ OCTOBER–DECEMBER (General Conditioning)

EMPHASIS	INTENSITY	REPS	SETS	REST INTVLS	TIMES/WEEK
gen. strength *(hypertrophy)*	70–80%	8–12	3–4	30–40 sec	3–4

* use for rest, injury or pleasure.

Chapter 9

Nutrition for Health and Vitality

Good health and personal accomplishments are determined by many factors including genetics, socioeconomics, culture, behavior and environment. Nutrition, too, plays a vital role throughout our life and it is one of the few environmental factors over which we have total control. For athletes and non-athletes alike, good nutrition can make all the difference between good and poor performance.

· For athletes and non-athletes alike, good nutrition can make all the difference between good and bad performance.

· Protein provides stamina, carbohydrates provide energy.

Athletes are generally presumed to be the epitome of health – both in their physique and their nutrition. Surveys have shown, however, that athletes eat food similar to that of the general population, only more of it! I see this trend regularly in my practice.

The nutritional demands on athletes make it imperative that they supply their bodies with foods that contribute to optimum health. The purpose of this chapter, then, is to provide the basic guidelines with which you can tailor your diet to your own needs and reap the rewards of health and vitality.

GUIDELINES FOR OPTIMUM NUTRITION

I. The seven key elements needed by the body are:

- uncontaminated water
- carbohydrates (complex and unrefined)
- lipids – commonly referred to as fats and oils (essential fatty acids)
- proteins (essential amino acids)
- vitamins
- minerals
- enzymes

Carbohydrates, proteins and fats are commonly called macronutrients because they must be consumed in large amounts in order to derive any useful energy. Vitamins, minerals and accessory nutrients which are essential for health in small amounts are called micronutrients. In order to maintain a healthy diet, you need to consume a suitable amount of these seven elements. In the past, specialists recommended that the macronutrients in your diet include seventy percent carbohydrates, fifteen percent proteins and fifteen percent fats (refer to Figure 9.1). The newest studies recommend that you eat forty percent complex carbohydrates, thirty percent proteins, and thirty percent fats (refer to Figure 9.2). In his book *In Fitness and In Health,* Philip Maffetone, offers compelling reasons for using the second approach: it helps to maintain stable blood sugar levels, it reduces fatigue and lightheadedness after physical exertion, it lowers the need to count calories, your mental and physical energy levels increase, and your metabolism works more efficiently.

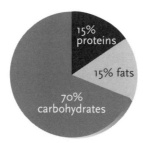

Figure 9.1 GENERAL RECOMMENDATION FOR DIETARY
COMPOSITION OF MACRONUTRIENTS

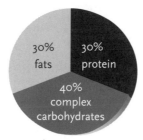

Figure 9.2 MAFFETONE'S RECOMMENDATION FOR DIETARY
COMPOSITION OF MACRONUTRIENTS

I recommend that the forty percent complex carbohydrates be taken in the form of whole grains such as brown rice, millet, quinoa, oatmeal, wholewheat cereals, potatoes, and a variety of beans such as chick peas, black beans and pinto beans. Refined carbohydrates such as pastas and breads should be ingested in moderation. Use the more refined carbohydrates only when quick energy is required and definitely not as the foundation of your diet.

2. *Digestion, assimilation and elimination.* If your digestion is efficient and you are eating "clean-burning" foods, your body will not have to work as hard to process the toxic by-products. This means the assimilation of nutrients will be greater.

The location of digestion depends on the type of foods eaten. For instance, only protein is digested in the stomach;

carbohydrates are digested in the mouth and small intestine, and fats in the small intestine.

To properly digest carbohydrates you must chew your food thoroughly so your body can prepare for the next digestive phase in the small intestine. If carbohydrate foods contain little or no protein they tend to move very quickly to the small intestine where their readily available energy is assimilated. If, however, they are mixed with protein foods, the process takes longer and energy availability is delayed.

When you eat proteins and carbohydrates separately, you speed up and improve your digestion. If your digestive system is sluggish or sensitive and you have a lot of gas after a complex meal then you should try eating your proteins and carbohydrates separately. Most people, however, could benefit from eating animal protein with low-carbohydrate vegetables. (Refer to the glycemic index chart later in this chapter for a list of low-carbohydrate vegetables.)

Fats and oils are digested and assimilated completely in the small intestine. The digestion of fats is a slow process and when fat-rich food is also high in protein, it can take as long as six hours to leave the stomach. You should remember this is when deciding what to eat before a race. The less the burden on your digestive tract, the more energy is available for performance. It is a good idea not to eat big meals late at night. The digestive system needs time to rest and the best time for this while you're sleeping. Finally, you should also avoid drinking liquids with meals as they will dilute your digestive enzymes.

3. *Avoid processed, nutrient-deficient "foods."* These foods deplete your body's vitamin and mineral stores when they are digested – sort of like having a hole in your car's fuel tank. As an athlete you cannot afford to let this happen. Certain additives and heavy metals in foods hinder the function of enzymes thus bogging down your body's natural vitality.

WATER

When you think that nearly seventy percent of your body is made of water, it's easy to understand that nearly every bodily function, from the transportation of nutrients to the elimination of toxins, happens in a liquid medium.

Fluids are the life source for everyone, and for the athlete adequate amounts of water are critical for optimum performance. In a recent study, a number of male athletes were made to take a treadmill test in which half of them were denied water while the other half were allowed to drink one cup of water every fifteen minutes. The study found that those who drank no water lasted about three-and-a-half hours while the other group were able to last seven hours! It is possible for you to lose up to eight pounds of sweat per hour during a strenuous sporting event and by the time you feel thirsty it is usually too late to avoid dehydration. During a race, then, you should drink about eight ounces (1 cup or 250 ml) of water every fifteen to twenty minutes. While you can survive a race without it, your recovery will be slower and you are likely to compromise your performance. Therefore, it is important to be proactive and keep yourself hydrated.

It takes very little fluid loss to affect you. Some research has indicated that even slight dehydration affects mental ability and muscular strength. When you lose around two percent of your body weight you will feel weak, your breathing will become harder and muscle fatigue will set in. At around four percent you feel very tired, a little lightheaded and your muscles feel heavy. At five percent or more your heart beats abnormally fast, you experience rapid breathing and you begin to lose your ability to concentrate. Fluid loss of more than six to eight percent will usually result in extreme dehydration and if not corrected could result in death.

Unfortunately, not all water is created equal anymore. Over the years many of our natural water supplies have been contaminated by acid rain, chemical leaching and industrial waste.

Today, the most common disinfectant used to treat drinking water is the inorganic mineral chlorine which reacts with naturally occurring organic compounds to form organohalides. This by-product is extremely mutagenic and carcinogenic for humans and animals. Studies have found possible associations between chlorinated water and cancer in the bladder, breast, colon and rectum. Other inorganic disinfectants such as alum and sodium fluoride cannot be used by the body and slowly build up in the system leading to such problems as kidney stones, arthritis and rheumatism.

Most experts agree that the purest water you can drink is distilled or "purified" water. Reverse osmosis filtered water is another wise choice as long as you make sure the filters are changed regularly and you have a good quality system. When you think of how much money you spend on your bicycle, shoes and other athletic equipment, an investment in good water will not only improve your athletic performance but your overall health as well.

And what about other beverages? Try to minimize – if not eliminate – the consumption of soft drinks with artificial sweeteners (e.g., aspartame); drink beer and wine in moderation and spirits sparingly, if at all. Coffee and tea remain controversial. Taken in moderation (one to two cups daily) they should pose no major problem. Keep in mind, however, that coffee and tea are diuretics, which will flush much-needed fluids from your body.

CARBOHYDRATES

Carbohydrates are the body's principal source of fuel. These nutrients provide us with calories that are immediately available as energy. Unfortunately, this easy source of energy can be quickly depleted when you work or train hard – the famous two-hour "bonk" for marathoners is the usual time it takes a trained athlete to deplete his or her carbohydrate stores. Although lipids and proteins can be used for energy, carbohydrates are the preferred source of fuel because of the ease with which they can be converted to energy. Athletes and younger children have faster metabolisms and so require higher levels of carbohydrates than most.

Carbohydrates are classified according to their structure: simple sugars (monosaccharides), two or more sugars (oligosaccharides) and complex carbohydrates (polysaccharides).

▸ *Monosaccharides* include glucose (e.g., dextrose, corn sugar, grape sugars), fructose (levulose, fruit sugar) and galactose. Food sources of monosaccharides include honey, fruit sugars and syrups.

▸ *Oligosaccharides* include sucrose, lactose and maltose. Examples of food sources include table sugar, beets and maple sugar.

▸ *Polysaccharides* include starches from beans (green, lima, kidney, navy), whole grains (such as brown rice, millet, barley, quinoa), wholegrain cereals (such as sugar-free granolas, seven-grain cereal), chick peas, tuberous vegetables, corn, leafy vegetables, noodles and potatoes.

▸ Fiber is also a complex carbohydrate that provides no energy or calories but is important in regulating the speed of bowel activity and for eliminating waste from the body.

HOW ARE CARBOHYDRATES USED BY THE BODY?

Carbohydrates are digested by the stomach and small intestine and then carried to the liver. From here they are used in one of five ways:

1. Many of the carbohydrates will be used for immediate energy needs.

2. Some will be stored as glycogen in the liver and tissues.

3. Some are converted to fatty acids and stored as triglycerides in fat tissue.

4. A small amount is converted to other necessary carbohydrates.

5. Some carbohydrates will become the carbon skeleton used for the production of non-essential amino acids.

If you are normally active and eat a diet high in natural complex carbohydrates you should not have to worry about the carbohydrates being stored as fat since these carbohydrates are a source of energy that is readily used up through regular activity. On the other hand, if you are sedentary and eat a diet of simple and refined carbohydrates such as those found in processed foods, you should worry about the carbohydrates being stored as fats. Processed foods made of refined sugar and flour, such as soft drinks and white bread, offer little nutritional value to the body.

If you eat an excess of simple carbohydrates you don't need to worry about excess fat but you may want to consider the effects this diet has on your general health. An overreliance on simple carbohydrates can cause overloads in blood glucose and possibly a deficiency of vitamin B1 (thiamine). This overload can also tax the adrenal glands and pancreas, causing them to work overtime in an effort to normalize your blood sugar level. Symptoms of blood glucose overload can range from mood swings to depression, anxiety, dizziness, blurred vision, insomnia and fainting. Ultimately this type of diet can lead to diabetes and adrenal exhaustion.

Adrenal exhaustion can also be brought on by the combined stresses of daily life, regular training and an excess of refined carbohydrates in your diet. I see this regularly in my practice among sedentary and active people. If this is not enough to make you curb your sweet tooth – consider this:

As you eat foods containing simple sugars, the body uses only those it needs and deposits the rest as fats and cholesterol. The deposits can be in the liver, heart, arteries, kidneys and muscles, and can result in conditions such as obesity, rheumatic disease, diabetes, tumors, liver and kidney diseases, and atherosclerosis. These fat deposits also reduce the oxygen level in the tissues thus slowing down your body's metabolism. This, in turn, causes fats to accumulate faster. When this happens all your exercise will seem to get you nowhere.

Eating Carbohydrates When in Training

BEFORE EXERCISE

Although "carbo-loading" is well known to most athletes, it is not well understood. The basic idea is to enrich your muscles' supply of glycogen. Here's how it works. Four to five days before a race, you increase your exercise load and eat a diet comprised of forty percent complex carbohydrates, thirty percent proteins, and thirty percent fats. The theory is that this will decrease the glycogen in the muscles and liver because of the increase in exercise. Then, two or three days before the race, you increase your complex carbohydrates to about seventy to seventy-five percent of your dietary intake, eating at least three big complex carbohydrate meals plus some proteins and fat over the next two or three days. This increases the glycogen stored in the liver and muscles. Glycogen is the stored form of glucose which is used by cells and tissues for energy. If your body requires more energy than the glycogen can provide, fat will be used. If your body fat is low, however, proteins in the tissues will be converted to energy. That's the theory – but does it work?

Interestingly, nothing in the current scientific literature supports the popular belief that a diet high in carbohydrates, particularly before a competition, improves athletic performance. In order for carbohydrates to have a positive effect on your performance, a healthy daily diet must be established over the long term. Many athletes have converted to the 40:30:30 ratio of complex carbohydrates : proteins : fats and they're finding that their performance has greatly improved. As always, experiment to find what works best for you.

DURING EXERCISE

In order to sustain performance over a long period it is advantageous to replenish carbohydrates on an ongoing basis. Heavy exercise depletes the muscles of glycogen. In fact, some researchers have found that athletes who train three or more hours per day actually never have a "full tank" because of the demands they place on their body. They usually require complex carbohydrates while training in order to compensate for declining levels of muscle glycogen. Eating carbohydrates can sometimes cause intestinal distress, so Dr. David Costhill recommends eating your pre-race/workout carbohydrates three hours beforehand. Since good hydration is critical to training or racing, it is best to consume these carbohydrates with water.

Once exercise begins, the minimum level of carbohydrates you need to maintain performance is around forty grams per hour of activity. This figure will vary according to your level of fitness and the intensity of your effort. Costhill recommends seventy to ninety grams per hour. You should experiment with these amounts so that you do not experience gastric distress. Too many racers have experienced serious problems because the only time they followed these recommendations was during a race. The body is already under stress during a race and unless it knows what is happening, it can (and usually does) experience some discomfort.

If you use energy drinks, the solution should contain five to ten percent carbohydrates to be effective. Drink one eight-ounce glass every fifteen minutes. In this way you will not tax your system and you will allow your body to maintain a stable level of carbohydrates.

Do not forget to drink water on top of any sports drink, otherwise you risk becoming dehydrated. For longer races, I always had two water bottles, one with water and the other with the "Power Mix," a carbohydrate, protein and flax oil mix (see recipe in Chapter 10). I would drink two bottles of water to every bottle of Power Mix. I also recommend adding the sports herbal formula Endurance® to your water bottle for more stamina.

AFTER EXERCISE

Replenishing glycogen stores after a workout is critical for speedy recovery and good hydration. Simple sugars can be safely taken at this point because it is a time when you need the quick energy these sugars can give. If you have a regular workout schedule but are not training hard, fresh fruit after exercise is a good way to balance your blood sugar level.

Table 9.1 RECOMMENDED CARBOHYDRATE INTAKE FOR ATHLETES

Body weight	Grams of carbohydrates per daily training hours					
KG (LBS)	2 HRS	3 HRS	4 HRS	5 HRS	6 HRS	7 HRS
40 (88)	200	300	400	500	600	700
50 (110)	300	400	500	600	700	800
60 (132)	400	500	600	700	800	900
70 (154)	500	600	700	800	900	1,000
80 (176)	600	700	800	900	1,000	1,100
90 (198)	700	800	900	1,000	1,100	1,200
100 (220)	800	900	1,000	1,100	1,200	1,300
110 (242)	900	1,000	1,100	1,200	1,300	1,400
120 (264)	1,000	1,100	1,200	1,300	1,400	1,500

Eat carbohydrates in small doses throughout the day to ensure optimum glycogen storage. These meals should consist of complex carbohydrates which are digested slowly. For the most part, avoid foods with a high glycemic index (over 82) such as honey, corn, white potatoes, instant grain cereals, white rice, raisins, white bread and other refined foods (see Table 9.2 below). These raise your blood sugar and insulin levels rapidly which is unhealthy. Instead, include a variety of vegetables, fruits, wholegrain pastas and breads, brown rice, yams and tofu in your diet. Nutritionally, these are superior foods.

GLYCEMIC INDEX

The glycemic index rates different foods according to the effect they have on your blood sugar level. This list was developed to help diabetics eat safely. The higher a food rates in the glycemic index, the more rapid will be the rise in blood glucose when the food is eaten, and this increases insulin production. A "good" food is one which has a low to medium glycemic index. Eating these foods will not cause a sharp rise in your blood sugar level. Please note that fructose (found in fruit) has a low glycemic value whereas most common breakfast cereals have very high glycemic values, often surpassing pure sugar (glucose).

Table 9.2 FOODS GROUPED BY GLYCEMIC INDEX

HIGH INSULIN INDUCERS

GLYCEMIC INDEX ≥ 100

corn flakes	rice cakes	puffed rice
puffed wheat	French bread	white bread (100)
tofu ice cream	maltose	glucose

GLYCEMIC INDEX 70–100

Grapenuts®	wholewheat bread	rolled oats
white rice	brown rice	muesli
shredded wheat	all-bran cereal	potato (russet)
potato (white)	mango	apricots
raisins	bananas	corn
kidney beans (canned)	corn chips	rye crisps
honey	ice cream	ice cream (low-fat)

MODERATE INSULIN INDUCERS

GLYCEMIC INDEX 40–70

pasta	oranges (also juice)	peas
instant potatoes	instant rice	chick peas
baked beans	navy beans	grapes
apples	potato chips	sucrose
lactose		

GLYCEMIC INDEX ≤ 40

wholegrain rye bread	oatmeal (slow cooking)	barley
black-eyed beans	lentils	kidney beans
lima beans	tomato soup	yogurt
milk	peaches	pears
plums	cherries	grapefruit
peanuts	fructose	

Healthy complex carbohydrates such as whole grains, fresh fruits and fresh vegetables should form the bulk of your dietary carbohydrates and you should keep to foods in the lower to moderate glycemic index range (forty to seventy percent and less than forty percent). When you are training intensely you can use more of the higher glycemic index carbohydrates (seventy to one hundred percent) and I would generally stay away from foods that rate less than 100 in the index.

FATS: TO EAT OR NOT TO EAT?

Contrary to popular belief, health and fitness depend to a large extent on having appropriate amounts of healthy fats in our diet. Unfortunately, this is one of the most misunderstood areas of nutrition. Even though research has shown that fats provide at least twice as much energy as carbohydrates, we have become afraid of fat because we know that seventy-five percent of the people in the industrialized world are killed by diseases of fatty degeneration. When I tell my patients to eat avocados or raw nuts and seeds, their response is usually, "Oh, but those are so high in fat." This is only part of the story!

Fats in our foods contain fatty acids which are involved in a wide variety of body functions. For example, fatty acids are required for energy storage and the absorption of vitamins A, D and E; they provide water barriers and insulation for cellular membranes and they produce chemical messengers that control cell growth, blood pressure, immune reactions and tissue inflammations.

Let's look at this a little more closely since all fats are *not* created equal. Fats and oils come in many forms. There are short-chain, long-chain, saturated, unsaturated, monounsaturated, polyunsaturated, essential and non-essential fats. Rather than go into a lengthy account about all the various compositions, we will simply highlight their key characteristics so that you can make an educated decision about which fats to use and which to avoid.

SATURATED FATTY ACIDS (SFAs)

The main building blocks of fats and oils are fatty acids. There are short- and long-chain saturated fatty acids. Short-chain SFAs are generally liquid at body temperature, partly soluble in water, easy to digest and are readily available for energy production in the body. Food sources of short-chain SFAs include butter, coconut oil and palm kernel fats. Long-chain SFAs are insoluble in water and are usually solid at room temperature. These fats are often related to diseases of fatty degeneration such as cardiovascular problems. Pork, beef and mutton tend to be high in long-chain saturated fatty acids. Remember, you don't have to eat saturated fats to have an overabundance of them in your body: refined sugars and starches are converted to SFAs so beware of these as well. While a certain amount of long-chain SFAs are necessary, you should monitor your intake as an excess can interfere with the functions of essential fatty acids and decrease metabolic rate and vitality.

UNSATURATED FATTY ACIDS (UFAs)

Unsaturated fatty acids are usually liquid at room temperature. UFAs include monounsaturated (MUFAs) and polyunsaturated (PUFAs). The most important MUFA is called oleic acid and is found in olive, almond and other seed oils, as well as in the fat deposits of most land animals. It stimulates bile flow and is the major fatty acid found in the secretion of skin glands. Studies show that people with a diet high in olive oil and low in butter have lower levels of cholesterol and lower blood pressure than those eating margarine and large quantities of butter. Olive oil fits into the "no harm" category but does not provide you with many essential fatty acids.

ESSENTIAL FATTY ACIDS: THE HEALTHY FATS

Essential fatty acids (EFAs) are extremely important in nutrition and health, yet these are the only fatty acids that are not manufactured by our bodies. As a consequence, they must be supplied through the diet. EFAs are known to reduce blood pressure, lower cholesterol and reduce the risk of blood clotting among a host of other benefits. They are also "essential" for building and repairing cells. Essential fatty acids in general ward off viruses such as herpes and influenza.

There are two categories of EFAs: omega-6 and omega-3. Omega-6 essential fatty acid, or linoleic acid, is abundant in evening primrose, safflower, sunflower, grape seed and almond oils (see Table 9.3). Signs of omega-6 deficiency might include eczema-like eruptions, hair loss, behavioral disturbances, susceptibility to infections, slow wound healing, sterility in males, miscarriage in females, arthritis, heart and circulatory problems and many other conditions.

Omega-3 essential fatty acid, or alpha-linolenic acid, is found in abundance in flaxseed oil, soybeans and walnuts, green leafy vegetables such as cabbage, spinach and broccoli, and fish such as herring, mackerel, sardines, tuna and halibut. Deficiency symptoms include growth retardation, physical weakness, vision impairment, learning disability, behavioral changes, tissue inflammation, water retention, dry skin, low metabolic rates, high blood pressure and sticky platelets associated with heart disease. You can reverse these by adding omega-3 essential fatty acid to your diet.

Fish oils are good sources of eicosapentaenoic acid (EPA), a member of the omega-3 family of fatty acids. These oils are important for the normal functioning of the brain cells, retinae, adrenal glands, sex glands and the nerve relay stations. Given the potential cost of fish, buy local and/or in-season fish or fresh frozen fish. Use other animal products (red meats, high-fat dairy products) in moderation.

Table 9.3 SOURCES OF ESSENTIAL FATTY ACIDS
Approximate percentage of total oil in nuts and seeds

OMEGA-6 ESSENTIAL FATTY ACID — LINOLEIC ACID

Almond oil (17%)	Peanut oil (29%)
Brazil nut oil (24%)	Pecan oil (20%)
Canola oil (30%)	Pumpkin seed oil (42%)
Evening primrose oil (72%)	Safflower oil (75%)
Flaxseed oil (14%)	Sesame seed oil (45%)
Grape seed oil (71%)	Sunflower seed oil (65%)
Hazelnut oil (16%)	Walnut oil (51%)

OMEGA-3 ESSENTIAL FATTY ACID — ALPHA-LINOLENIC ACID

Canola oil (7%)	Pumpkin seed oil (15%)
Flaxseed oil (58%)	Soy oil (9%)
Poppy seed oil (30%)	

PROCESSING OF OILS

The most harmful stage of oil processing is hydrogenation, a means of hardening oils into solids. In this procedure the oil is saturated with hydrogen atoms by mixing it with a metal catalyst and then subjecting it to high pressure and temperatures as high as 385°F (196°C). The molecular structure of the hydrogenated oils (margarine, shortening and other oils often used in baked goods, ice cream, candy and snack foods) has been so radically altered that it is unrecognizable and unusable by the body. The oil is physically and chemically changed and forms trans-fatty acids which are potentially carcinogenic and disrupt normal metabolism of essential fatty acids.

Commercial oil production uses temperatures ranging from 200–500°F (93–260°C). This destroys enzymes and other natural nutrients and makes more trans-fatty acids. Don't let the commercially produced oils labelled "cold-pressed" fool you –

even these oils are subjected to tremendous heat from friction generated by the giant screw presses. Because no external heat is applied, commercial processors can legally label these oils cold-pressed. For your health, choose *expeller-pressed*, unprocessed oils. Extra-virgin olive oil is the one exception to this rule. While it is not expeller-pressed, the oil can be safely extracted from the olives without heat and therefore without harm. If possible, choose oils in dark, glass bottles which protect against spoiling from light.

You can offset the effects of trans-fatty acid-rich diets by consuming high levels of beneficial fatty acids found in expeller-pressed oils such as canola (stay away from European brands), extra-virgin olive, flaxseed, sesame, soy and fish oils. Vitamin E also helps alleviate the negative effects of "bad" oils. In Holland trans-fatty acids have been banned while in North America it is estimated that some "food" goods have as much as sixty percent trans-fatty acids in them.

You may well ask, "If I'm not supposed to heat oils, how do I cook with them?" Some oils offer more heat stability than others. Use sesame oil, cocoa butter and butter when cooking at low heats. If the oil becomes black or brown while cooking, throw it out and start again at lower heat. For baking, these oils are too strong in taste so I use butter instead. Although it will end up being heated in the process, you can lessen the negative effects by cutting back the butter in the recipe by one half and substitute a similar amount of fresh fruit purée or yogurt to maintain consistency and texture. For cold foods such as salads, or for adding oil to soups and pasta after cooking, I use a blend of extra-virgin olive oil and flaxseed oil.

BUTTER VS. MARGARINE

When I think about the subject, it seems unlikely that natural saturated animal fats, which humans have been consuming since time immemorial, have caused the abrupt rise in incidents of heart disease since 1900. Nevertheless, there is a correlation between the rise of heart disease and the replacement of the butter churn, olive press and expeller-pressed oils with industrial oil refineries.

Margarine contains diacetyl, isopropyl and steryl citrates, sodium benzoate, benzoic or citric acid, di- and monoglycerides, and many other chemicals. No healthy margarine is available – it doesn't matter whether it says it is polyunsaturated or not. A natural, solid polyunsaturated fat at room temperature does not exist – it has to have been chemically altered by hydrogenation and totally denatured to get that way. Butter, on the other hand, is a saturated fat in its natural state.

Choose butter over margarine. Butter is more easily digested than margarine. Butter contains healthy fatty acids, vitamins and minerals.

As athletes must use fuel efficiently, avoid eating long-chain saturated fatty acids, refined and hydrogenated fats. Stay away from oils exposed to light (through transparent bottles), refined heated oils, fried and deep-fried oils, margarines, shortenings and partially hydrogenated oils. Finally, moderate your intake of the saturated fats in pork, beef, mutton and dairy products.

EAT BUTTER WITHOUT GUILT!

Mix together:
1 cup (240 g) of butter (room temperature)
1 cup (240 ml) of flaxseed oil or olive oil
Store in the refrigerator.

I use this combination when I make popcorn, it tastes great and I can eat more! Use it whenever you would use butter – this way you are getting some essential fatty acids and at the same time you are reducing your intake of saturated fats. So you don't ever have to feel guilty about using butter.

CHOLESTEROL: THE GOOD, THE BAD AND THE MISUNDERSTOOD

There are "good" cholesterols and "bad" cholesterols. For most people good cholesterol does not exist and many athletes are unnecessarily preoccupied with their cholesterol intake. It is, however, a vital material in the human body. For example, cholesterol produces the bile acids that digest fats and it is a major component of brain and nerve tissue. The body makes hormones from cholesterol, which allow for glucose synthesis and suppression of inflammations. Cholesterol should not comprise a large part of your diet because your body manufactures most of the cholesterol you need from sugars, fats and proteins. The more harmful fats you consume, however, the greater is the pressure on your body to make cholesterol. A greater problem occurs when cholesterol-rich foods are exposed to air; then the cholesterol is targeted by free radicals and if you eat these foods cell damage can occur.

Where does bad cholesterol come from? Overcooked meats, smoked or aged meats, dairy products and overcooked eggs. (Eggs are not bad for you if you do not overcook or oxidize (fry) them. Boil eggs and keep the yolk soft to reduce the formation of cholesterol oxides. Eggs do not increase your blood cholesterol levels because they contain lecithin which emulsifies the cholesterol in them.) Homogenized milk does more damage to arteries than eggs or meat ever will as the fat globules have been mechanically manipulated to be so small that they can be readily and directly absorbed into the bloodstream.

Cholesterol travel throughout the body by means of protein molecules called lipoproteins. There are two main types of lipoproteins in the body: high-density lipoproteins (HDLs) and low-density lipoproteins (LDLs). HDLs are often called "good cholesterol" because they remove excess cholesterol from the tissues. The low-density lipoproteins (LDLs) carry cholesterol –

from the liver to the bloodstream and to the cells. It is the ratio of HDLs to LDLs that determine good health. Whether or not you are a competitive athlete, I recommend you have lipid-panel blood tests done to determine your cholesterol levels and your ratio of LDLs to HDLs.

Very few people are aware of the difference between dietary cholesterol and blood cholesterol. Dietary cholesterol comes from food and blood cholesterol is made by the body and found in the bloodstream. Eating foods containing dietary cholesterol will not necessarily put cholesterol into the bloodstream. However, eating a food with "no cholesterol" but which contains palm oil or coconut oil (which are very high in saturated fats), will elevate blood cholesterol levels.

PROTEINS

Next to water, proteins are the most plentiful substance in the body. Proteins form muscles, organs, glands, bones, teeth, skin, hair, enzymes and hormones. Without proteins in our diet, the building and repair of all body tissue would be impossible. Many athletes and coaches have mistakenly assumed that they should consume excessive quantities of protein because of its vital role in building and repairing the body. Proteins *do* repair the body *and* provide energy, but you need not consume vast quantities of protein-rich foods to achieve this end. Rather, you should focus on eating moderate amounts of foods that combine complementary amino acids (the building blocks of all proteins) on a daily basis. Only in this way will you get the most repair, growth and energy out of your diet.

Amino acids are grouped into two categories: *essential* and *non-essential*. You must supply essential amino acids in your diet. Animal proteins are considered *complete proteins* since they supply all essential amino acids while vegetables, grains, nuts and seeds are considered less complete because they only supply some of them. This does not imply in any way that vegetables and grains are less desirable protein sources. If you take care to consume a proper mix of legumes, grains and nuts you can be sure you are getting a full complement of essential amino acids.

Plant sources of the essential amino acids (in italics) are as follows:

▶ *Isoleucine.* Baked beans, cashews, pumpkin seeds, papaya, avocado, olives, brown rice and eggplant.

▶ *Leucine.* Same sources as isoleucine.

▶ *Lysine.* Beans, most nuts, apples, apricots, pears, grapes, bananas, carrots, beets, turnips, alfalfa and brewer's yeast.

▶ *Methionine.* Lentils, soybeans, barley, rye, corn, millet, oats, Brazil nuts, pineapple and dates.

▶ *Phenylalanine.* Soybeans, sweet potatoes, most greens, beets, carrots, most nuts, oats and pumpkin seeds.

▶ *Threonine.* Most nuts, brown rice, peaches, bananas, green leafy vegetables, yams and asparagus.

▶ *Tryptophan.* Pumpkin seeds, barley, rye, oats, dates, strawberries and most vegetables.

▶ *Valine.* Mushrooms, almonds, sesame seeds, corn, millet, pomegranates, apples, dandelion greens, okras, parsnips and tomatoes.

You do not need to combine all essential amino acids at the same meal. The body has the ability to store essential amino acids and you can draw upon them as your needs dictate. You simply need to eat a variety of foods that will provide the full complement of aminos. Choose from the following list to ensure that, when eaten together, your foods provide a full complement of all eight essential amino acids.

▶ *Grains + Legumes.* Rice and bean casserole, wheat/soy bread, lentil curry on rice, corn/soy bread, bean or pea curry on rice, baked beans and wheat bread, corn tortillas and beans, legume soup with bread.

▶ *Grains + Milk Products.* Cheese bread, pasta with cheese, rice/milk pudding, barley and yogurt soup.

▶ *Seeds + Legumes.* Sesame salt on legumes, sesame seeds in bean soups, hummus (sesame paste and chick pea spread), sunflower seeds and peanut mix.

▶ *Grains + Seeds.* Rice with sesame or sunflower seeds on top, breads or muffins with sesame or sunflower seeds, any grain with added seeds.

▶ *Legumes + Milk Products.* Legume soups with milk, cheese and beans.

If you are a vegetarian who does not combine amino acids to form complete proteins, you will feel fine for a while as the missing amino acids will be provided by the body's protein pool. Eating the same incomplete proteins all the time, however, results in amino acid deficiencies at a cellular level. If you eat a complete complement of amino acids, your body will not have deficits. Amino acid supplements are discussed in Chapter 11.

TIPS FOR OPTIMUM PROTEIN USE

▶ Eat protein early in the day and not for your evening meal.

▶ Eat complete amino acid groupings.

▶ Do not combine dairy protein with any other kind of animal protein.

▶ Avoid refined carbohydrates.

▶ Eat smaller, simpler meals.

▶ Do not eat protein with sugar or sweets of any kind.

▶ Do not drink liquids at your meals.

▶ Eat protein with a variety of vegetables.

▸ Eat protein with good quality oils.

▸ Take proteins as a meal, not as a snack.

▸ Make the protein in nuts and seeds easier to digest by soaking them overnight in water, draining them, then storing them in the refrigerator.

▸ Minimize high-stress proteins such as red meat, milk, raw nuts and seeds, soybeans and pork. (High-stress proteins are not readily usable by the body and create toxic waste that must be removed by the kidneys.)

▸ Exercise regularly, if modestly.

By eating foods high in carbohydrates you avoid toxicity problems but you are not eating what your body tissues require. Tissue is built from protein and a steady stream of carbohydrates will weaken the tissues. To maximize tissue health, choose high-protein vegetarian sources (see Table 9.4) and eat high-stress proteins in moderation. Remember, protein provides stamina, carbohydrates provide energy. When you heal slowly it's often a sign of protein deficiency at a cellular level.

Those of you who want to pay closer attention to the ratio of protein, carbohydrates and fats in your diet should refer to Figures 9.1 and 9.2. Note that there is also a moderate to high level of protein in some common carbohydrate foods (e.g., spelt, quinoa or soy). You do not necessarily have to consume more animal protein to maintain higher protein levels.

Table 9.4 PROTEIN VALUES OF VARIOUS FOODS
Protein in grams per 100 g (3 oz) portion

PLANTS

FRUIT

All fruit (0.2–2)

VEGETABLES

Carrot (1)	Cabbage (1)	Cauliflower (3)
Broccoli (4)	Kale (4)	Parsley (4)
Brussels sprouts (5)		

GRAINS

Rice (7)	Barley (8)	Corn (9)
Rye (9)	Millet (10)	Buckwheat (12)
Oats (13)	Red wheat (14)	Spelt (15)
Amaranth (16)	Quinoa (18)	

NUTS AND SEEDS

Hazelnuts (13)	Almonds (19)	Sesame seeds (19)
Sunflower seeds (24)		

LEGUMES

Adzuki beans (22)	Dry peas (24)	Lentils (2)
Soybeans (35)		

FERMENTS

Amasake (3)	Tofu (8)	Miso (15)
Tempeh (20)		

ALGAE/SEAWEEDS DRIED

Hijiki (6)	Kombu (7)	Wakame (13)
Kelp (16)	Dulse (22)	Nori (35)
Chlorella (55)	Blue–green algae (60)	Spirulina (68)

YEAST

Nutritional (50)

ANIMAL PRODUCTS

DAIRY

Milk (whole) (3)	Yogurt (9–15)	Cottage cheese (14)
Cheese (25–31)		

FISH

Oysters (9)	Clams (14)	Herring (17)
Cod (18)	Bass (18)	Abalone (18)
Anchovies (19)	Mackerel (19)	Sardines (24)
Tuna (29)		

MEAT AND EGGS

Eggs (3)	Fowl (16–24)	Beef/red meat (17–21)
Beef heart (20)	Beef liver (20)	Chicken liver (21)

ENZYMES — NATURE'S POWERHOUSES

Enzymes are energized protein molecules that regulate all bio-chemical activities in the body. One of their principal functions is to initiate the oxidation of glucose, which creates energy for the cells. Enzymes are also essential for food digestion, stimulation of the brain and repair of all organs, tissues and cells.

The two most potent enzymes in the body are the digestive enzymes *amylase* and *protease* which break down carbohydrates and proteins, respectively. The pancreas secretes digestive juices containing high concentrations of amylase and protease along with another enzyme called *lipase* for digesting fats. Enzymes ingested in your food and secreted by the pancreas and stomach are hard at work when you eat and digest. When you eat hurriedly or in a stressful environment, enzyme secretion is compromised and your digestion is poor. Chew, chew, chew — eat slowly to ensure adequate enzyme secretion.

All live, fresh or whole natural foods contain enzymes so be sure to get lots of raw fruits and vegetables in your diet. The fresher and more vital the food, the more constructive the enzymes and the more able they will be to reduce stress on the body. The longer the food's growth cycle has been interrupted the more the enzymes are destroyed. Raw juices are an excellent source of highly concentrated vital enzymes, assuming they are drunk shortly after juicing. Certain fermented foods such as fermented juices, sauerkraut, yogurt and tempeh are also high in enzymes.

Eating well is important for good health, and this is largely a matter of common sense. A properly balanced diet will include all the macronutrients as well as the micronutrients, which we will examine in Chapter 11. But first, let's see how we can get the most energy out of our diet.

Chapter 10

Eating for Energy

According to a Statistics Canada report, Canadians are now spending more time in hospitals than they were in the 1970s. While this is due in part to an aging population, many of our health problems can be linked to a lack of basic nutrition. Every stage of food production affects food quality therefore there are many ways to improve or diminish the nutrient levels in the foods we eat. As shown below, the nutritional benefits in food can be destroyed by the time they get to your shopping cart, so it makes sense to find out as much about your food as you can before you buy it.

· Every stage of food production affects food quality, and food quality affects your health and your ability to perform.

· If your body is constantly breaking down toxic substances, the energy available for mental and physical performance is compromised.

▶ *Soil.* The condition of the soil is the most important factor in determining the quality of our foods. Many soils today are depleted by commercial nitrogen fertilizers which increase crop yield but do nothing to improve the soil's nutrient content. Chemical fertilizers will deplete iron, zinc and other trace minerals from the soil.

▶ *Chemical Agriculture.* Pesticides, herbicides, growth hormones and antibiotics used in farming cause health problems in humans. These toxins accumulate in the fat cells of animals, and if you consume animal products you will ingest a higher concentration of these chemicals which will in turn be stored in your fat tissue. Toxins not only have potential long-term health risks but also undermine your health in the short term. If your body is constantly attempting to break down and excrete these toxic substances, the energy available for mental and physical performance is compromised.

- *Harvesting.* Careless and premature harvesting can take a toll on nutrient levels in foods. Today fruit and vegetables are often picked long before they are ripe. Consider a tomato that is picked green and ripened in storage: it has been calculated that the level of vitamin C alone will be reduced by eighty percent.

- *Storage.* Foods that are shipped long distances and stored for long periods of time – sometimes under fluorescent lighting – will lose nutrients. Now we have the recent development of "irradiated" foods that will not spoil. This process exposes food to radioactive materials like cesium-137 and cobalt-60 to prevent sprouting and to kill bacteria, mold and fungi. Another miracle? Or a nutritionist's nightmare? A 1984 study by Ralston Scientific Services for the US Army found that mice fed a diet rich in irradiated chicken died earlier and had a higher incidence of tumors.

- *Preservatives.* To prevent spoilage, food has always been mixed with other ingredients such as herbs, salt and spices, but in the past thirty to forty years there has been a steady increase in the chemicals added to foods. For example, there are 1,200 legal additives for ice cream! One of the emulsifiers used in place of eggs in certain commercial ice cream brands is diethyl glycol which is a component of antifreeze and paint remover. The wonderful vanilla flavor is from piperol which is used to kill lice and if cherry is your favorite flavor you will likely be ingesting acedaldehyde C-17 which is used in plastic and rubber cement. Over 3,000 different chemicals are being used in commercially grown foods!

▸ *Food Processing and Refining.* While a moderate amount of food processing is necessary today, it is nevertheless the single greatest destroyer of nutrients. In some cases, nutrients are added back to refined food, but certainly not in the way nature intended.

Our North American idea of "basic" foods includes pizza, sugar-laden snacks, burgers, fries, dairy products, coffee, muffins, soda pop – all of which are actually non-foods. We wonder why we are generally fatigued and not feeling well, and why our children have allergies, learning disorders, chronic colds and ear infections. The fact is we can only look forward to these conditions developing into more chronic, serious diseases as we get older – unless we start eating real foods.

ORGANIC FOODS

The term "organic" refers to the method of raising plants and animals without the use of chemical fertilizers, pesticides, growth hormones or other additives. Instead, crop rotation, animal or green manures, organic soil amendments and other non-toxic means are used by organic farmers to keep the soil fertile to cultivate natural foods. Organic products contain little or no chemical residue and offer a high nutrient value.

If you eat whole foods and eliminate (or at least dramatically reduce your consumption of) "non-foods" you will decrease the total toxic burden on your body, and, if you make great demands on your body, you need to seriously consider how you fuel your system.

CLEANSING

Given the multitude of poisons that affect our lives, it is difficult
to expect our bodies to stay healthy, especially when we demand
increased athletic performance. The integrated approach to
health includes cleansing – a natural way to rid your body of
toxins and reduce your exposure to the environmental pollutants found in foods.

In colder climates the ideal time to cleanse is in the spring
or early summer. In the winter the body is under stress because
of the cold weather and so will have greater metabolic demands
than in warmer seasons. I encourage my patients to cleanse at
least once a year, however I do not recommend water fasting for
anyone, particularly as an initial cleanse. I usually recommend
the cleanse in four-week stages.

WEEK 1

► Eat *only* fresh fruit and vegetables, either raw or steamed.
  Choose two to three whole grains to eat on a rotating basis
  such as millet, brown rice and quinoa. You may eat unlimited
  amounts of these foods.

► Eat raw seeds in moderation. Natural herbs such as parsley,
  oregano, celery, garlic and ginger can be used for seasoning. A
  minimal amount of sea salt is fine but I would recommend
  seaweed over salt.

► Drink at least four eight-ounce glasses of fresh organic vegetable juice daily.

► Completely avoid all animal products such as meat, chicken,
  fish, eggs and other dairy items.

► Completely avoid coffee, caffeinated teas, alcohol and tobacco.

► I recommend homeopathic remedies to detoxify the liver and
  kidneys, and psyllium and bentonite to cleanse the bowels.

- Do not use any vitamin or mineral supplement, with the exception of vitamin C, during any stage of the cleanse.

WEEK 2

- Consume only fresh organic vegetable and fruit juices during the second week. Drink a minimum of six eight-ounce glasses of freshly made juice and at least eight glasses of water with fresh lemon daily.
- Continue using homeopathic remedies, psyllium and bentonite.

COMING OFF THE CLEANSE: WEEKS 3 AND 4

Once you have completed Week 2 you should follow with three to five days from Week 1. Nuts, seeds, whole grains, beans and "good" oils should be added slowly in the first five to seven days after Week 2. Finally, proteins such as meat, fish, yogurt, eggs and cheese can be incorporated into your diet in Week 4. Eat only one portion of animal protein daily in Week 4.

ENERGY BARS

Energy bars may be handy food substitutes but if you are going to choose one, read the label carefully and then let your taste buds make the final decision. Some energy bars taste like flavored dental adhesive while others, when cold, require a hacksaw to cut through and taste like rich syrup. Although we have never been big fans of these items, when used wisely and sparingly, they can provide a better alternative to junk food and can get you through a long workout. Then again, a recent study by researchers at Ball State University in Muncie, Indiana found that when a group of endurance-trained male cyclists was given bagels and another group fed energy bars, there was no difference in their athletic performance or respiratory exchanges after a one-hour bike ride. So, while energy bars may contain a few extra vitamins and cost more than a bagel, their popularity may be more related to marketing hype than to performance enhancing characteristics.

If you do eat power bars, you should avoid those that contain hydrogenated vegetable oils, sugar, peanuts and peanut butter, aspartame and any artificial ingredients and preservatives. Prefer instead those that contain dried fruits, seeds, whole grains, honey, malt syrup, rice syrup, soy protein and nuts other than peanuts.

ENERGY DRINKS

If your training includes hard sessions of more than seventy-five minutes, you will likely deplete your blood glucose and muscle glycogen, and so any carbohydrates you consume before the workout will be used for energy. Sports drinks (and bars) are formulated to meet both your fluid and energy needs. Under strenuous exercise conditions, water simply does not do it!

The common carbohydrate sources are fructose, sucrose, maltodextrin, corn syrup, glucose polymers and polylactate. Concentrations of carbohydrates per eight-ounce serving range from five percent in Carbo Gold® to ten percent in Performance® (maltodextrin and fructose): Coca Cola® contains twelve percent carbohydrates using corn syrup and fructose. Calories per serving can range from 41 (Carbo Gold®) to 100 (Performance®). Orange juice has around 112 calories.

Another important element of sports drinks is their sodium concentration. Dehydration can disturb the electrolyte balance that is essential for all bodily functions. Sports drinks replace any sodium lost through perspiration. Sodium also stimulates thirst and can delay urine production, which, depending on your point of view, may be helpful or troublesome during exercise. The amount of sodium varies considerably between sports drinks. Carbo Gold® has 5.4 mg of sodium per eight-ounce serving, while Gatorade® has 110 mg. Try several to determine which is best for you.

By regulating the fluid balance inside and outside the cells, electrolytes are necessary for muscle contraction, relaxation and general muscle metabolism. An imbalance of the minerals (chlorine, potassium and sodium) which become electrolytes in the body can lead to early muscle fatigue and a corresponding drop in performance. For an athlete, the muscles may feel "great," but they just won't respond to the demands you place on them. This is one reason electrolyte replacement drinks are so popular among athletes. It is essential that the drink be taken *before* the event to "preload" the system and then consumed at intervals during the event.

Which drink is best? It is largely a matter of taste but you might want to consider these basic guidelines when purchasing energy drinks.

- Glucose polymer is the easiest on the stomach and it can move out of the stomach faster than water.
- An eight-ounce serving should contain between twenty and twenty-eight grams of carbohydrates for maximum benefit.
- Drinks should contain the key electrolytes such as potassium, calcium, sodium, chloride, magnesium and phosphates.
- Avoid drinks which contain sucrose.
- Fructose and maltodextrin are easily absorbed by the digestive system.
- Avoid all drinks which contain any artificial flavors, colors, etc. They have no ergogenic benefits.
- Consume the drinks slightly chilled, if possible, as this allows for better absorption.
- Remember you must always drink beyond your thirst.

Experiment with a variety of these products to determine which is best for you – just be careful of your overall sugar and carbohydrate intake.

BASIC RULES OF FOOD COMBINING

The premise of food combining is that you should eat combinations of foods that take the same amount of time to digest, thereby ensuring optimal digestion. Sugars in the form of fruit and fruit juices digest very quickly, with refined carbohydrates running a close second. Complex carbohydrates are also quickly digested and assimilated if not combined with fats or proteins. Proteins, on the other hand, take up to six hours to digest and fats even longer. So, if you eat an animal protein (which also contains fat) with a glass of fruit juice, the fruit juice will digest immediately, the protein and carbohydrate will ferment and the enzymes needed for protein and fat digestion will be inhibited by the fermentation process. One of the worst combinations I can think of is the typical North American breakfast: a glass of orange juice, eggs, bacon and toast or hash browns – look out stomach!

Although food combining can get very complex, these simple rules are easy and they'll get you started on the road to optimum digestion.

► Eat fruit separately from all other foods (allow one hour for digestion). The exception to this is cooked fruit (e.g., jams and preserves) as the enzymes will have been destroyed by cooking which means there will be less fermentation if eaten with proteins and fats. Sometimes you can get away with combining fruit with carbohydrates as both are digested fairly quickly.

► Keep animal proteins and carbohydrates separate.

► Never eat more than one animal protein at the same meal.

► Eat melons alone, or leave them alone.

MENU SUGGESTIONS FOR ATHLETES IN TRAINING

Note that items marked with an asterisk (*) are contained in the recipe section later in this chapter.

BREAKFAST

Fresh vegetable juice* every morning

Monday: Mixed grain granola with yogurt or soy milk

Tuesday: Oatmeal with maple syrup and soy milk

Wednesday: Quinoa with Oats* and apple sauce

Thursday: Millet-Raisin-Apple Porridge* with cinnamon and maple syrup

Friday: Kasha Cereal* served with rice syrup or maple syrup

Saturday: Quick Brown Rice Pudding*

Sunday: 7-Grain Cereal with rice milk or soy milk

MORNING SNACKS

If you work out in the morning, eat fresh fruit after the workout. Then an hour later have a snack such as:

- raw nut-and-seed mix with dried fruit (optional)
- soy milk drink
- amasake drink
- Blender Drink Mix*
- Almond Milk*
- yogurt and fruit
- congee*

Note: Any of these drinks can be added to your breakfast or lunch for added calories and protein.

LUNCH

I am assuming that most people eat lunch in restaurants. I recommend that you bring your own lunch to work, but as this is not always possible, please consider the following lunch suggestions. Choose your restaurants carefully and ask for extra vegetables and made-to-order meals if they don't have what you want. Try to find restaurants that use extra-virgin olive oil (Greek and good Italian restaurants are usually pretty reliable).

Monday: Animal protein such as chicken, fish or meat with lots of mixed steamed vegetables

Tuesday: A hearty bean soup with a large salad

Wednesday: Omelet with large salad and steamed vegetables

Thursday: Vegetable pasta dish with salad

Friday: Chinese stir fry with no MSG

You can see that I am making recommendations that do not combine animal protein and high carbohydrates such as rice or potatoes. If you find you are getting hungry a couple hours after lunch (a sign of good digestion), you may want to slow the digestive process a little by eating a carbohydrate (e.g., rice, wholewheat bread or corn bread) with the meals that contain an animal protein. If you get hungry by mid-afternoon then take a high-quality snack food to work rather than grabbing some fast non-food. Eat your protein meals without carbohydrates and snack if you are hungry between meals.

Try to eat the majority of your food, particularly proteins, during the earlier part of the day and keep to smaller portions for the evening meal. This takes a bit of adjustment but it will give the digestive system a break while you are sleeping. Eating a large meal later in the evening doesn't allow your digestive system to rest and so you probably won't sleep as well, nor will you wake up feeling refreshed.

AFTERNOON SNACKS (*around 3–4 PM*)

Eat lighter snacks in the afternoon and if you must snack in the evening, keep it very light (e.g., fruit).

- muffins – the wholegrain and high-fiber variety containing nuts and seeds
- cookies such as oatmeal with nuts or seeds
- nuts and seed mix (soaked in water) with sprouts
- wholegrain, high-fiber bread with sesame spread or butter
- baked corn chips with guacamole
- leftovers
- congee*
- hummus*
- miso soup (a simple mix of miso paste and water)
- any of the morning snacks

DINNER SUGGESTIONS

Monday: Amaranth Pilaf with Almond Béchamel Sauce*

Tuesday: Pasta with your choice of sauce, vegetables and salad

Wednesday: Barley/Soybean Loaf*

Thursday: Scalloped potatoes made with soy milk (substitute soy milk for cow's milk and use a mix of soy cheese and cheddar cheese) accompanied by steamed vegetables

Friday: Baked Quinoa, Sunflower Seed and Vegetable Loaf*

Saturday: Festive Wild Rice*

Sunday: Sushi with miso soup and salad

RECIPES

Quinoa with Oats *(serves 2–4)*

1 cup quinoa, soaked in water	1 cup rolled oats
3 cups water	1 tsp sea salt

Rinse quinoa several times before soaking. Place all the ingredients in a 2-quart pot, cover and bring to a boil. Reduce heat to low and simmer 30 minutes. Turn off heat, let sit 5 minutes before serving.

Millet-Raisin-Apple Porridge *(serves 2)*

1 cup millet, soaked	3 cups water
few grains of sea salt	1 apple, cut up
1 cup raisins	

Rinse the millet several times before soaking. Place all the ingredients in a pot, cover and bring to a boil. Reduce heat to low and simmer 30 minutes. Serve with cinnamon and soy milk on top.

Kasha Cereal *(serves 2–4)*

1 cup buckwheat groats	few grains sea salt
4–5 cups boiling water	1 cup figs or raisins

Place all the ingredients in a pot. Bring to a boil, reduce heat to low and simmer 30 minutes until groats are soft.

Quick Brown Rice Pudding

2 cups leftover brown rice   1 cup raisins
cinnamon to taste   maple syrup to taste

Mix the ingredients in a bowl. Serve with sesame seeds or sunflower seeds, and rice or soy milk on top. This can be warmed up if you like, but it is also good cold.

Blender Drink Mix

1 cup soy milk   1 banana
1 cup water   1 cup frozen strawberries
1 tbsp nutritional yeast (optional)   1 tbsp chlorella or spirulina

Mix the ingredients in a blender until smooth. This drink does break the rules of food combining but most people can digest it well.

Power Mix

3 tbsp protein powder (*I recommend rice as the source of protein*)
1 water   2 tsp expeller-pressed flax oil

Mix the ingredients in a glass. Stir well. You can carry this energy drink in your water bottle on longer rides or runs.

Almond Milk

3 cups hot water   1/2 cup blanched almonds
4 tbsp honey, if desired

Purée all ingredients then strain the mixture through cheese-cloth or a fine strainer. Discard the strained almond pieces. For a richer drink you can add more almonds.

Congee

1 cup rice (or millet, spelt or any other grain)
6 cups water

Mix one cup of rice into six cups of water. Cook the rice and water in a covered pot for 4–6 hours over a very low heat. Note that it is better to use too much water than too little, because the longer congee cooks, the more "powerful" it becomes.

Eaten throughout China as a breakfast food, this simple rice soup is easily digested and assimilated, provides energy, aids digestion and is very nourishing. In Chinese medicine, rice is known to strengthen the digestive center.

Hummus

3 cups garbanzo beans (chick peas)
2 (or more) large cloves garlic, finely minced
5 tbsp lemon juice
1/4 cup tahini (sesame butter)
1/2 tsp soy sauce or more to taste

Soak the beans overnight. Drain the beans and cover them with fresh water. In general, you should use five times as much water as beans. Bring to a boil then simmer 2–3 hours, or until the beans are tender. Drain the liquid from the beans and set it aside. Blend the ingredients until you have a spread with the consistency of mayonnaise. If the hummus is too thick, add some liquid from the beans. Top the hummus with a little olive oil and serve with raw vegetables or bread. Refrigerate any leftovers in a covered container.

Amaranth Pilaf with Almond Béchamel Sauce *(serves 6–8)*

1 small onion, minced	1 tsp oil (optional)
1 cup amaranth	2 cups bulgur wheat
1 tsp sea salt	7–8 cups boiling water
3/4 cups lentils, soaked in water for 40 minutes	

Sauté the onion in a large (4–6 quart) pot over moderate heat. Turn down the heat and stir in the amaranth, bulgur and lentils. Add the salt and boiling water. Cook the mixture for 30 minutes, stirring occasionally. Pour the mixture into a casserole dish and cover it with the almond sauce (see below). Bake at 375°F (190°C) for 15 minutes.

Almond Béchamel Sauce

2 tbsp oil	4 tbsp flour
1/2 cup almonds	1 tbsp mint
2 cups water, almond or other nut milk, heated	
Seasoning: sea salt, miso, soy sauce or a dash of nutmeg	

Heat the oil in a heavy saucepan. Stir in the flour, whisking for 1–2 minutes. Remove the flour from heat, add the liquid and stir until the mixture is smooth. Return the sauce to heat, add the seasonings and bring the mixture to a boil. Reduce heat and simmer the sauce until it is thick. Stir in the almonds and mint before serving.

Barley/Soybean Loaf *(serves 4–6)*

3 tbsp sesame oil	1 cup soybeans, cooked
1 cup barley, cooked	1 tomato, cut in small pieces
1 carrot, diced	1/2 tsp sea salt
1 carrot, grated	1 bay leaf
1 turnip, sliced	1/2 green pepper, diced
1 cup mushrooms	2 free range eggs
1/2 cup olives	garlic and onions optional

Grease a medium-sized casserole dish with the sesame oil. In a bowl, mix together all the ingredients except the olives. Pour the mixture into the casserole dish and top with the olives. Bake the loaf at 375°F (190°C) for 25 minutes.

Baked Quinoa, Sunflower Seed and Vegetable Loaf *(serves 4)*

3 cups cooked quinoa
1 cup flour (wholewheat, barley, etc.)

1/2 cup warm water	1 tbsp miso
1 tbsp lecithin granules	1 tsp each basil and thyme
1 onion, chopped	2 cups carrots, sliced
1 cup broccoli, cut	2 tbsp sunflower seeds, dry roasted
parsley	

Lightly oil a 2–3 quart baking pan. Combine the quinoa and flour in a bowl. Set aside. In a large bowl, dissolve the miso and lecithin in warm water. Add the herbs to the quinoa-flour mixture until well combined. Steam the onions, broccoli and carrots for 7 minutes. Gently add the vegetables to the quinoa "dough." Place the loaf into the baking pan. Sprinkle with sunflower seeds. Bake the loaf at 350°F (175°C) for 30–40 minutes. Serve garnished with parsley.

Festive Wild Rice *(serves 6)*

1 cup long-grain brown rice	1 cup wild rice
1/2 cup pine nuts	6 cups water
1/2 cup mushrooms, sliced	1/2 cup onion, diced
1 lb (454 g) tofu, cubed	2 tbsp soy sauce
1/2 tsp each basil and thyme	parsley for garnish

Wash the rice carefully, draining off any impurities and excess water. Set aside. In a skillet or in the oven, dry roast the pine nuts until lightly browned. Combine the rice and water in a 3-quart casserole dish. Layer the remaining ingredients over the rice. *Do not stir.* Cover and bake at 350°F (175°C) until the water has been absorbed, about 1–1 1/2 hours. Garnish with fresh parsley and serve.

Favorite Juice Recipes

The following fresh juices can be easily made using a good-quality juicer. Remember to drink these juices right away so that their precious nutrients aren't lost.

GINGER COMBO

4–5 carrots
1/2 inch of fresh ginger

1/2 apple

GARLIC PLUS CLEANSER

4–5 carrots
1 small beet
1–2 large garlic cloves

spinach
1 stalk celery

CALCIUM COCKTAIL

3–4 large kale leaves
large bunch of parsley

4–5 carrots

POTASSIUM REPLENISHER

large handful of spinach
medium-sized bunch of parsley
2–3 stalks celery
2 red potatoes
2–3 carrots

Note: You can drink the potato juice separately if you don't like it mixed with other juices.

TIPS TO MAXIMIZE HEALTH AND MINIMIZE EXPOSURE TO ENVIRONMENTAL TOXINS

- Eat foods in the most natural, unprocessed form possible.
- Buy only organic dairy products, grains, beans, meats and produce.
- Avoid non-organic produce from countries where pesticide standards are lax (e.g., Mexico and Spain).
- Avoid processed, "non-foods" (white sugar, white flour and chemical-laden foods).
- Eat slowly and in a relaxed atmosphere.
- Buy and store foods in glass containers instead of plastic.
- Avoid chlorinated water and drink a minimum of eight to ten glasses of good water daily.
- Use only expeller-pressed, unrefined oils.
- Perform a cleanse at least once a year.
- Safeguard your health with vitamin and mineral supplements.
- Have your home checked for electromagnetic field disturbances – these should be avoided.
- If you spend long hours at a computer, use protective screens (e.g., those that have anti-radiation, anti-glare and anti-static qualities).
- Buy unbleached paper products.
- Avoid showering or swimming in chlorinated water.
- Use biodegradable cleaning supplies with no bleach.
- Use natural fabrics in clothing, bedding and furniture.
- If you live in an urban area try to make regular visits to the countryside or mountains for some clean air.

The foundation for optimal health is based on pure, wholesome foods, clean water, clean air, sunlight, exercise, rest and relaxation, stress reduction and a positive mental attitude. This was the code of the "nature cure" doctors in the late eighteenth- and early nineteenth centuries. It sounds pretty basic, doesn't it? It is easy if we work with the proper tools, even though these tools may be scarce.

Naturopathic medicine is founded on the time tested *principal vis medicatrix naturae* – the healing power of nature. Today more than ever, nature needs our help just as much as we need nature to augment our personal health. If we destroy our environment, we eventually destroy ourselves. This is a biological law. If we protect our environment it will nurture us and provide for us.

In the past two chapters we have covered a great deal of the essential foods needed to properly fuel our bodies. Even so, our diet may not provide all the vitamins, minerals and other nutrients we require, especially if we are training a lot. We will round out our examination of nutrition with a discussion about vitamin and mineral supplements.

Chapter 11

The ABCs of Vitamins and Minerals

So much has been written about nutritional supplements that the average person is often at a loss to know which supplements, if any, will benefit their health. Add to this confusion the fear of trying something "controversial" and the result is that many people shy away from using supplements. What most people fail to understand is that while supplements may not always be categorized as official ergogenic aids, this does not mean they cannot enhance your performance.

· Supplemental vitamins and minerals, when combined with proper diet and training, can bring about marked improvements in your strength, speed and endurance.

· A lack of any one of the important minerals can lead to disease.

Optimum nutrition can maximize the body's physiological and biochemical functioning but it cannot extend your physiology beyond its hereditary limits. Supplemental vitamins and minerals, when combined with proper diet and training can, however, bring about marked improvements in your strength, speed and endurance.

Deciding which supplements to take can pose a daunting challenge to even the most experienced athlete, and so this chapter will be devoted to providing a balanced and informative survey to help you understand the "ins and outs" of supplements. We will review the essential vitamins and minerals and provide general guidelines for using them. If you choose to follow any of these guidelines, you should first consult with a qualified health practitioner who is trained in dietary supplementation and the specific needs of athletes.

Studies show that certain mineral deficiencies can be responsible for headaches, anxiety, fatigue, depression and nervousness, among a variety of other emotional and physical disorders. In fact, ample evidence shows that poor nutrition plays a major role in premature aging and the disease process. When you subject your body to the additional stress of training, you must supply the proper amount of vitamins, minerals and supplements needed by your system. By themselves, they will not make you go faster or get stronger but they will enhance your health and general behavior.

GETTING FULL COVERAGE

The Recommended Daily Allowance (RDA) is a guideline developed by the Canadian and American Food and Nutrition Board for the adequate intake of essential nutrients like vitamins and minerals. The guidelines are minimal and are meant only for normal, healthy people. Supplements may be necessary if you have a dietary deficiency or are training hard.

The best way to ensure you get full coverage with your supplements is to take a multivitamin and multi-mineral complex which supplies all the vitamins and minerals in small doses (to prevent deficiencies), then use additional single vitamin or mineral supplements in higher doses according to your needs and goals. There are powdered forms of supplements on the market for those of you who don't like to swallow pills.

ANTIOXIDANTS

One of the best ways to maintain the body's state of generative health is through exercise which supplies oxygen to the cells.

Strenuous exercise, however, will increase free radicals in the body and it is for this reason that you should incorporate antioxidant supplements into your diet. Free radicals are highly reactive molecules which can cause cell damage. However, they are not always bad. Normally, free radicals are present in the body in small amounts to fight disease, produce vital hormones and to activate enzymes. When too many free radicals are created in the body, however, cell damage occurs. Antioxidants are substances, usually vitamins, minerals or enzymes, that prevent oxidative damage and protect against free radicals. For example, lemon juice, which contains

DOSES

Doses for vitamins, minerals and other supplements are commonly given in:

· milligrams (mg)

· micrograms (mcg)

· International Units (IU)

Most doses are given by weight, that is, milligrams or micrograms. The exceptions are vitamins A, D, E and beta-carotene, which are measured by their biological activity and expressed in International Units. For example, one IU of vitamin E could contain 0.91 milligrams of dl-alpha tocopherol or it could contain 0.67 milligrams of d-alpha tocopherol or even 1.12 milligrams of dl-alpha tocopherol succinate, all of which are different sources of vitamin E.

vitamin C, is an antioxidant and is used to prevent apples from turning brown, that is, oxidizing. In a similar way, antioxidants can be used to prevent oxidative damage in the body.

Free radicals are produced by normal body metabolism, exposure to radiation and environmental pollutants. Healthy cells have an enzyme coating that protects them from the degenerative effects of oxygen. These enzymes are catalase, reductase, superoxide dismutase and glutathione peroxidase. Unhealthy cells and disease microbes do not have these coatings so oxygen is able to attack them and create free radicals. Antioxidants include the vitamins A, C and E, the carotenoid beta-carotene, the minerals zinc and selenium, and the bioflavonoids.

Do not let this discussion of antioxidants lead you to believe that too much oxygen is bad for you. *Hypoxia, or lack of oxygen, in the tissues is the fundamental cause of all degenerative diseases.* The best way to optimize health is to oxygenate every cell in the body. The more oxygen you have in your system, the more energy you produce and the more efficiently you eliminate waste products.

The presence of free radicals in your body can lead to tissue damage and diminished energy production. Evidence suggests that free-radical damage contributes to the beginning of chronic conditions and degenerative diseases such as cancer, cardiovascular problems, emphysema, arthritis, osteoporosis and cataracts.

SOURCES OF FREE RADICALS

- fried foods
- cooked saturated fats and oils
- nitrates and nitrites in meats
- breathing toxic chemicals
- cigarette smoke
- exposure to radiation
- strenuous exercise
- chlorinated water
- high-fat diets

ATHLETES' REQUIREMENT OF ANTIOXIDANTS

Strenuous exercise greatly increases free radical production due to increased secretion of catecholamines from the adrenal glands. If you are training less than one hour daily at fifty percent of your maximum heart rate you have a low antioxidant need. If you are training one to two hours at seventy percent of your maximum heart rate you have a medium antioxidant requirement. If you are training more than two hours a day you have high antioxidant needs. Those of you with "low" needs should take the minimum recommended dose; those with "medium" needs should take a dose midway between the minimum and maximum, and those with "high" needs should take the maximum recommended dose.

Vitamins

WHAT ARE VITAMINS?

The vital amines, or vitamins, were discovered at the turn of the century and are defined as carbon compounds that cannot be synthesized by our bodies but which are needed in small amounts. There are twenty vitamins that are important in human nutrition and they fall into two categories: fat-soluble vitamins such as A, D, E and K; and water-soluble vitamins such as B and C. Water-soluble vitamins are more easily absorbed by the body than fat-soluble vitamins but they are more easily lost through sweat and urine. If you are physically active, you may need to supplement your diet with water-soluble vitamins.

Vitamins have many important functions, including:

- assisting essential chemical reactions
- regulating your metabolism
- converting fats and carbohydrates to energy
- forming bones and tissues
- preventing deficiency diseases
- providing antioxidant protection against free-radical damage and environmental toxins

VITAMIN A AND BETA-CAROTENE

Vitamin A strengthens your immune system and protects mucosal tissues. Vitamin A and beta-carotene (a precursor to vitamin A, also called provitamin A) prevent stress-induced thymus atrophy, can actually promote thymus growth and maintain smooth, soft, disease-free skin. Beta-carotene belongs to a powerful antioxidant family called carotenes. Carotenes are found in plants while vitamin A is found only in animal sources. Vitamin A is fat-soluble and is not readily excreted from the body whereas beta-carotene is water soluble. Beta-carotene must be converted to vitamin A before it can be used by the body.

Some people prefer to take beta-carotene instead of vitamin A because beta-carotene can be consumed in large amounts without signs of toxicity. Some of the early signs of toxicity are headaches and fatigue. If you are drinking a lot of carrot juice and supplementing with beta-carotene your skin may turn orange. Not to worry, the beta-carotene is merely being stored in the tissue – just reduce your intake for awhile.

Recommended dose: Vitamin A 10,000–20,000 International Units (IU), although it should be avoided during pregnancy. Beta-carotene 25,000–50,000 IU daily.

Food sources: Green leafy vegetables, carrots, sweet potatoes, yams, apricots, cantaloupe, broccoli and squash.

B VITAMINS: THE ANTISTRESS VITAMINS

All B vitamins are water soluble and must be constantly replenished since they are not stored in the body. They play an important role in providing the body with energy by assisting in the conversion of carbohydrates into glucose, which the body burns to produce energy. Let's briefly review the individual components that make up B-complex vitamins. (Note: I recommend taking a mega B complex (this contains all the B vitamins at approximately 50 mg each) as general support. Should you want to take any of the single B vitamins, take them in addition to the mega B, otherwise you will become deficient in the other B vitamins).

B1: THIAMINE

Thiamine is called the "good disposition" vitamin because it is important in maintaining mental well-being. It is essential in carbohydrate metabolism and in the synthesis of acetylcholine (the nerve hormone that makes muscles move). Chlorinated water, alcohol, caffeine and sulphites destroy thiamine. Thiamine deficiency is very common even at the conservative RDA levels, and a USDA study of 38,000 people found that forty-five percent of the study group had a thiamine deficiency. Thiamine is not known to be toxic even when taken in large amounts.

Recommended dose: 50–100 mg daily.

Food Sources: Brewer's yeast, torula yeast, soybeans, brown rice, sunflower seeds, peanuts and whole wheat.

B2: RIBOFLAVIN

Vitamin B2 is crucial for energy production and is involved in the regeneration of glutathione – one of the main cellular protectors against free-radical damage. Even moderate exercise in females increases riboflavin requirements. Vitamin B2 in foods is easily destroyed by light but not by cooking. When you start taking vitamin B2 (alone or in a multivitamin) your urine can turn a bright yellow-green color, a normal occurrence and nothing to worry about.

Recommended dose: 50–100 mg daily.

Food Sources: Organ meats (kidney, liver, heart); almonds, mushrooms, whole grains, soybeans and green leafy vegetables.

B3: NIACIN

Niacin-containing enzymes play an important role in energy production; they help metabolize fat, cholesterol and carbohydrates and they manufacture many body compounds such as adrenal hormones. Niacin plays a role in the glycogen energy cycle and so athletes' niacin requirements are higher. Studies have shown that megadoses of niacin can speed up glycogen use.

Recommended dose: 30–100 mg daily.

Note: Some people find their skin flushes after taking niacin. This only lasts a short period and is in no way dangerous.

Food sources: Liver and other organ meats; eggs, fish and peanuts (these foods are also rich in tryptophan which is converted by the body to form niacin). Plant sources of niacin include legumes, whole grains (except corn), avocados, rice and wheat brans, peanuts, brewer's and torula yeasts.

B5: PANTOTHENIC ACID.

Pantothenic acid is very important for athletes, since it supports the adrenal glands (see Chapter 14) which are taxed in all athletes. B5 is necessary to convert fats and carbohydrates into energy, and for the manufacture of steroid hormones and brain neurotransmitters. This vitamin does have positive ergogenic effects.

Recommended dose: 200–400 mg daily.

Food sources: Whole grains, legumes, sweet potatoes, broccoli, oranges, strawberries, liver, fish and poultry.

B6: PYRIDOXINE

Adequate B6 intake is crucial to maintain hormonal balance and a strong immune system. It is active in blood production, central nervous system metabolism, and amino acid metabolism. It follows that the more proteins (amino acids) you eat, the more B6 you will require.

Recommended dose: 30–60 mg daily.

Food sources: Whole grains (not flours), legumes, bananas, seeds and nuts, potatoes, Brussels sprouts and cauliflower.

B12: CYANOCOBALAMIN

If you are a vegetarian you should watch your B12 levels as this vitamin is mainly available from animal sources. Factors affecting B12 levels are listed below:

▶ Excessive intake (greater than forty percent of your dietary intake) of refined carbohydrates such as meat and other animal products can more than double your B12 requirements.

▶ Drugs and beverages such as alcohol, caffeine and nicotine, to name a few, will destroy B12.

▶ Oral contraceptive use.

▶ Low thyroid function.

▶ Intestinal parasites.

▶ Vitamin C supplements taken in doses higher than 500 mg will destroy fifty to ninety-five percent of B12 in the food if taken at the same time.

▶ Egg albumin and egg yolk decrease B12 absorption and a twenty percent soy bean drink increases fecal excretion of B12. Therefore, you should consider taking B12 supplements if you eat these foods frequently.

Recommended dose: 5–10 mcg daily. Vitamin B12 is best absorbed sublingually (under the tongue).

Food sources: Mainly animal products – organ meats, eggs, cheese, seafood and red meats. It is also found in fermented foods like brewer's yeast and in sea vegetables like kelp and nori.

BIOTIN

Biotin helps your body manufacture and metabolize fats and carbohydrates. This vitamin is made in the intestines by gut bacteria. Don't eat raw egg whites as they contain avidin which binds biotin and prevents its absorption.

Recommended dose: 100–300 mcg.

Food sources: Cheese, organ meats, eggs, mushrooms, cauliflower, soybeans and nuts.

FOLIC ACID

Folic acid is needed for healthy red blood cells and for brain and nervous system function. Various studies show a widespread folic acid deficiency in North Americans. The current RDA is extremely low for athletes and so it is a good idea to have your folate levels checked.

Recommended dose (assuming you have no current deficiency): 800 mcg daily. If you have a deficiency, increase the dose to 1,200–1,600 mcg daily and retest after three months.

Food sources: Green leafy vegetables such as kale, spinach, beet greens and chard; legumes, asparagus, broccoli, root vegetables, black-eyed beans, peas, brewer's and torula yeasts.

VITAMIN C

Vitamin C is a very versatile antioxidant and when combined with other antioxidants such as vitamin E, the effect of both is improved. Vitamin C is water soluble, therefore it has a special role as an extracellular defense against free radicals such as those that attack the lungs and brain during strenuous exercise. Its primary function is the manufacture of collagen, which is an important protein for structures that hold our body together (connective tissue, cartilage and tendons). Vitamin C also protects against free-radical damage caused by pollution, a very important function these days.

I often hear of athletes who catch a bad cold or flu after a major competition. Vitamin C is antiviral and antibacterial and its main effects are to boost the immune system, increase interferon levels, improve antibody responses, white blood cell function, thymus hormone secretions and connective tissue integrity.

Proof in the pudding? Double Nobel Prize winner, Dr. Linus Pauling, was often ridiculed during the early 1970s when he recommended mega doses of vitamin C. His critics often said such "excesses" produce little more than expensive urine. His research suggested quite the opposite, that somewhere along the evolutionary trail we lost the genetic codes to make vitamin C in our bodies, thus developing a need to ingest it. The fact that he outlived virtually all his critics (he lived to be nearly 100) may be a testament to the importance of vitamin C.

Recommended dose: I usually recommend 3,000–5,000 mg daily unless this causes flatulence or loose stools. In that case cut back to bowel tolerance level, that is, the highest dose of vitamin C you can take without getting diarrhea. After you have determined your tolerance level, adjust the dose so that you experience no discomfort. Some people can take up to 12 g daily without gastric distress. But don't try high levels of vitamin C in ascorbic acid form as it will likely cause problems even at low levels. The best forms are the ascorbates or ester-C.

Food sources: Vitamin C is found in abundance in vegetables such as broccoli, peppers, potatoes, Brussels sprouts, kale, parsley, collard greens, turnip greens and, of course, citrus fruits. But don't be fooled by the amount of vitamin C allegedly contained in these foods (e.g., 60 mg of vitamin C in an orange); most fruits and vegetables are picked long before we eat them and are then stored under fluorescent lighting – both of which readily destroy vitamin C. Most of us need to supplement our diet with vitamin C.

VITAMIN E

When shopping you'll notice there are different forms of vitamin E on the market: d-alpha tocopherol (natural source) and dl-alpha tocopherol (synthetic) and dl-alpha tocopherol succinate. Vitamin E is the best-documented fat-soluble antioxidant vitamin, and taken together with selenium works synergistically to combat oxidative stress.

Controlled studies on athletes given large doses of d-alpha tocopherol showed improved muscle performance, endurance and speed of recovery as long as the treatment was maintained. Avoid taking vitamin E and iron supplements at the same time of day. Any inorganic form of iron such as iron sulphate can impair the absorption of vitamin E. The more polyunsaturated fatty acids you consume in your diet, the greater will be your need for vitamin E.

Recommended dose: 400 IU twice daily.

Food sources: Raw nuts and seeds, whole grains, avocados, green leafy vegetables, tomatoes and berries.

Other Supplements

CHOLINE

Choline is required for the proper metabolism of fats and is very beneficial for lowering cholesterol levels. If you are eating a high-fat diet for caloric reasons you should consider taking choline supplements. Choline is most commonly available as choline bitartrate, citrate or chloride, or the form phosphatidyl-choline which is found in lecithin.

Recommended dose: 350–500 mg daily.

Food sources: Egg yolks (primarily phosphatidylcholine), liver, soy, cauliflower and lettuce.

COENZYME Q10

Coenzyme Q10, sometimes called the miracle nutrient, plays a central role in energy production. This ergogenic aid strengthens the heart muscle and energizes the cardiovascular system. It also stimulates insulin, stabilizes blood sugar levels and has antioxidant properties.

Recommended dose: 100–150 mg daily.

Food Sources: Coenzyme Q10 is available in every plant and animal cell, however supplements are required to produce beneficial effects.

GLUTATHIONE

Glutathione peroxidase is an enzyme formed from glutathione (a protein produced in the liver) and selenium. It protects the lung tissue from oxidative stress during exercise. Glutathione levels in the muscles and liver drop sharply when you exercise to the point of exhaustion.

Recommended dose for athletes: 200–400 mg daily.

PROANTHOCYANIDINS

These bioflavonoids are very powerful antioxidants. They are found in foods such as blueberries, grapes, fruits, some nuts and vegetables, but the supplement forms (which are highly concentrated) come from Maritime pine tree bark or grapeseed extracts.

The grapeseed proanthocyanadins cross the "blood brain barrier," a system designed to protect the brain and connective tissue from aging. This transporting ability of grapeseed offers additional antioxidant protection. Grapes belong to the antioxidant group called polyphenols.

Studies reported in *The Lancet* show that mortality rates from coronary heart disease decreased when high levels of flavonoids were taken. Proanthocyanidins are fifty times more powerful than vitamin E and twenty times more powerful than vitamin C in their ability to offset oxidative damage.

Recommended dose: 150–200 mg daily.

Food sources: The white part beneath the skin of citrus fruits, berries, onions, parsley, legumes, tomatoes and green tea.

AMINO ACIDS

An overview of amino acids is given in Chapter 9 under the heading *Proteins*. This section specifically addresses amino acid supplements.

A question I often hear is: "Do I have to eat meat to get my amino acid complement?" The answer is *no*. In general, for those who prefer not to eat meat, I recommend a complex amino acid supplement either in tablet form or as a protein drink. If you choose a drink, choose one that has an easily digestible base such as rice powder or soy. Soy protein is harder to digest, so if you have a sensitive digestive system, it is best to stick to the rice-based amino acid drinks.

SINGLE AMINO ACIDS

Canadian readers should note that single amino acids are not readily available in Canada. If you are interested in taking aminos you could use a complex vitamin supplement instead, or contact my clinic (403) 228-1907 for a list of US sources. Some experts claim that single amino acids taken over long periods can create amino imbalances. Because the long-term effects of taking single amino acids are unknown, please consult with an expert before adding them to your diet. If you do decide to take single amino acids, take them in cycles with "breaks" in between – even if you are taking complex amino acids in conjunction with single amino acid supplements. The best source of amino acids, however, is from whole proteins as your body is used to getting them in this form.

ARGININE

Arginine boosts the immune system, detoxifies the liver, helps increase muscle mass and lowers body fat. It is also good for arthritis and connective tissue disorders.

Recommended dose: I am basing these recommendations on research done at the Colgan Institute:

► 5–15 hours of training per week, 130–170 lb (59–77 kg): 4–8 g; 170–220 lb (77–100 kg): 9–16 g.

► 16–24 hours of training per week, 130–170 lb (59–77 kg): 5–10 g; 170–220 lb (77–100 kg): 12–20 g.

Food sources: Meats, gelatin, peanuts, chocolate, corn, cashews, almonds and peas.

CARNITINE

This is not an essential amino acid but it can be synthesized by the body from another amino acid called lysine. Carnitine is very important for providing energy to the muscles, particularly the heart. It also speeds the liver's oxidation of fats thereby increasing available energy. The energy is stored as adenosine triphosphate (ATP) which is used in muscle contraction. Muscle carnitine levels increase with exercise, and carnitine improves stress and exercise tolerance in animals. Daily use of carnitine results in significant improvements in cardiovascular function in athletes. Carnitine also improves stamina and energy metabolism within the muscles.

Recommended dose: There are different forms of carnitine but the most widely available, and least expensive, is L-carnitine. Take 2 g of carnitine two to three times daily. In Canada, all forms of carnitine are available by prescription only.

Food sources: The best source of carnitine is red meat but chicken, fish and cheese have small amounts as well. Vegetarians get little or no carnitine in their diet without taking supplements.

CREATINE

Creatine is made of several amino acids. It can be synthesized by the liver, kidneys and pancreas and then is used mainly by the skeletal muscles. Muscle creatine decreases significantly in high-intensity, short bouts of exercise and only decreases a little following sustained endurance exercise. Creatine is a good ergogenic aid if you are a swimmer, cyclist, sprinter or if you are involved in an explosive action sport. Creatine monohydrate (the most easily absorbed form of creatine) appears to be more beneficial if you are training and have already developed significant muscle mass. On the other hand, it may not be very effective if you are not in training.

Recommended dose: Creatine monohydrate, 5–7 g taken with water after workouts.

Food sources: Creatine levels are highest in herring, salmon, tuna and red meats. Vegetarians often have no creatine in their diet and therefore have lower levels of creatine in their muscles.

GLUTAMINE/ORNITHINE

During exercise the muscles release larger quantities of the non-essential amino acid glutamine than any other amino acid. This loss must be made up from other amino acids. In one significant study, 40 "overtrained" athletes were compared to 40 "well-trained" athletes. Plasma concentrations of glutamine were lower in the overtrained athletes. Those who took amino acid supplements did *not* have a drop in blood glutamine levels after strenuous exercise. Glutamine levels are definitely affected by long- and short-term muscular stress. Furthermore, a definite relationship exists between overtraining and weakened immune systems when the body's glutamine levels are depleted. Taking amino acid or glutamine supplements will keep your immune system strong.

The best form of glutamine for supplementation is in the form of ornithine alpha-ketoglutarate which is a glutamine substrate. Pure glutamine breaks down into ammonia which definitely interferes with performance. But alpha-ketoglutarate contains no ammonia – in fact it acts as an "ammonia scavenger" along with ornithine. Ornithine will more easily release growth hormones if it is used in conjunction with arginine or alpha-ketoglutarate. Take ornithine alpha-ketoglutarate and arginine hydrochloride three hours away from other amino acids and other protein foods.

I suggest taking single amino acid supplements in cycles of eight to ten weeks with rest breaks of four to six weeks in between.

Recommended dose: Ornithine alpha-ketoglutarate should be taken in the following doses:

- 5–15 hours training per week, 130–170 lb (59–77 kg): 2–4 g; 170–220 lb (77–100 kg): 4.5–8 g.

- 15–24 hours training per week, 130–170 lb (59–77 kg): 2.5–5 g, 170–220 lb (77–100 kg): 6–10 g.

Arginine hydrochloride doses are generally twice the amount recommended for ornithine alpha-ketoglutarate. If glutamine is taken individually, I recommend a dose of 500–1,000 mg three times daily.

GLYCINE

Glycine has been shown to release growth hormones which cause muscle growth. Injection of glycine in doses as small as 4 g can cause the release of growth hormones and a daily dose of 6 g of oral glycine can raise growth hormone levels fourfold. A study from the Princeton Brain Bio Center showed that a daily dose of 30 g taken orally can raise growth hormone levels tenfold. Be careful not to take glycine before a hard workout as it can give you a bad headache.

Recommended dose: 5–10 g daily.

MINERALS

Most North Americans' diets are deficient in minerals, and a lack of any one of the important minerals can lead to disease. Every cell in your body needs minerals as they enable your body to perform all its functions, from blood clotting to nerve transmission to muscle contraction. They are also necessary for your body to properly use vitamins and other nutrients.

Farmlands have been stripped of minerals over the past hundred years and so they produce foods that are also mineral deficient. For example, studies show that corn grown in soil mineralized with glacial gravel (organic fertilizer) had 57% more phosphorus, 90% more potassium, 47% more calcium, 60% more magnesium and close to 9% more protein than corn grown with chemical fertilizers.

BORON

Boron is essential for the manufacture of such steroid hormones as testosterone and 17-beta estradiol (a form of estrogen). In a group of postmenopausal women, one group was given estrogen and other given boron: the group given boron were able to assimilate calcium better. Boron deficiency may contribute to the high rate of osteoporosis in North America as boron helps your body assimilate calcium. Most North Americans do not get enough boron in their foods.

Recommended dose: 2–3 mg daily except during periods of intense exercise, for which I recommend taking 3–6 mg daily.

Food sources: Fruits and vegetables are the main sources if there were adequate amounts of boron in the soil in which they were cultivated.

CALCIUM

Calcium is important for the stabilization of enzyme systems, blood clotting, nerve transmission, muscle responsiveness and it provides the mineral matrix for bones and teeth. Many people, however, feel that if we just throw calcium at the bones, it will stick. Not so. Calcium needs many other vitamins and minerals such as magnesium, boron, manganese, phosphorus and vitamin D in order to be efficiently absorbed. Your body's hydrochloric acid levels must also be adequate for efficient absorption of calcium.

Numerous studies have shown that athletes do not get enough calcium in their diet. Exercise increases bone mineralization and increased bone density means you require more calcium. Female athletes are at an even greater risk of calcium depletion than men because strenuous exercise affects their hormones and ability to assimilate calcium. It is not unusual for a female athlete to develop amenorrhea (loss of periods) which is a good indication that calcium is lacking. When you look at a list of foods high in calcium, you must remember that only forty percent of the dose you take is actually assimilated by the body. Therefore, you must calculate the calcium levels of the food you eat and then supplement accordingly to maintain appropriate levels for your sex and age.

Recommended dose: 1,200 mg daily. Athletes, however, require extra calcium. In Canada the recommended dose indicated on the label refers to the amount of *elemental calcium* (amount absorbed), however, in the US, the dose refers to the *total amount of calcium*. Be aware that there are different absorption rates for the various calcium sources. Don't assume that if a label reads 1,000 mg calcium lactate that you will assimilate

OSTEOPOROSIS

Osteoporosis is a concern for all women, not only female athletes. Over 5 million spontaneous fractures occur a year – two-thirds of those in women and one-third in men. An x-ray is not a reliable test to determine loss of bone mass because thirty to fifty percent of a person's bone mass must be lost before any abnormality shows up. It is important to note that calcium deficiency is not the only cause of bone thinning.

Some of the other factors contributing to osteoporosis include increased phosphate sources in the diet (from animal proteins and junk foods, for example). The normal ratio of phosphorous to calcium should be 1:1 whereas most people have ratios between 2:1 and 4:1 thus causing excessive calcium excretion. Other "bone busters" include vitamin C deficiency, a sedentary lifestyle, alcohol, high salt and sugar intake and high levels of toxic metals in the body. Your body's toxic metal levels can be determined by hair analysis.

For men and women, wild yam cream or herbal preparations are good natural progesterone precursors.

1,000 mg of calcium. For calcium lactate you will absorb only 14% of what you ingest, calcium citrate 30%, calcium acetate 32%, calcium gluconate 9%, calcium carbonate 39% and from milk 27%. I don't recommend taking bone meal, as it can contain high levels of lead, nor do I recommend taking oyster shell, which can contain many contaminants as well.

Rethink your coffee habit. Caffeine drains calcium from your body, thereby weakening the bones. Another study showed that if you drink one cup of coffee each day you increase your risk of getting a hip fracture by sixty-nine percent. Those who took calcium supplements had a greater bone density even though they drank coffee. Caffeine also affects magnesium and sodium excretion.

Food sources: Kelp, tofu, kale, turnip and green leafy vegetables; soy milk, molasses, almonds, carrot juice, buckwheat, dandelion greens, Brazil nuts, goat's milk, sunflower seeds, sesame seeds, carob, brewer's yeast, figs, dulse and of course dairy products. You may want to reconsider the place of dairy products in your diet. For example, kale has ten times the amount of calcium as a similar-size portion of milk.

CHROMIUM

Chromium is a trace mineral essential for the metabolism of carbohydrates and amino acids and for the synthesis of cholesterol, fats and proteins. It is necessary for energy and maintaining stable blood sugar levels. Studies at the USDA Human Nutrition Research Center show that aerobic exercise results in significant chromium use and excretion: after a six-mile run chromium losses were one-fifth of pre-run levels and on exercise days chromium losses doubled. This deficiency is compounded in athletes who consume lots of sugar and refined carbohydrates. In another USDA study, those subjects whose diets were high in simple sugars showed chromium losses of up to 300 percent.

Recommended dose: 400–800 mcg daily. The best source is a chromium-niacin complex with high biological glucose tolerance factor (GTF). In the body, the GTF is responsible for the proper use of glucose.

Food sources: Foods that are high in chromium are brewer's yeast, organ meats, fish, poultry, whole grains, breads, cheese, nuts and dried fruits whereas fresh fruits, vegetables and dairy products have low concentrations by comparison.

IRON

Iron is essential to every cell in the body, but according to the World Health Organization, iron shortage is the most common dietary deficiency in the world! Basically, iron carries oxygen around in the body and is used in the formation of new red blood cells (which contain hemoglobin). Even a ten percent drop in iron levels can affect athletic performance. How much iron do you need? *Do not follow the RDA.* The first thing is to have your iron status assessed through blood work – but, do not measure just hemoglobin levels – they could be completely normal, while you could still be extremely iron deficient. Measure serum ferritin levels to see how much iron you have stored in your body. You may also want to have your folic acid and B12 levels checked at the same time.

If levels are low then you should take supplements over and above the recommended doses listed here. If levels are normal then you need to assess how much iron you use and gauge your intake accordingly. Most sedentary people use 1.0–1.5 mg of iron daily. Athletes require more because of increased perspiration; the more you sweat the more iron you lose.

Endurance athletes sweat 44 oz (1.3 litres) of fluid per hour and lose about 0.5 mg of iron per hour when in training. If you are working out for three hours or more, you can lose iron at a rate of more than than 1.5 mg per hour. There is conflicting information about the rate of iron loss through hemolysis (red blood cell breakdown) as runners' feet repeatedly hit the ground. I frequently see hemolysis in athletes and treat it with iron supplements.

Recommended dose: I usually recommend that male athletes supplement their diets with approximately 35 mg of iron daily and female athletes approximately 40 mg daily through foods when possible or supplemental liquid iron or tablets.

The actual amounts of iron required by the body are approximately 3.5 mg daily for males and 4 mg daily for females, but only ten percent of the iron you take in is absorbed. Unless you use one of the Floradix® products, iron supplements should be taken with food and vitamin C.

According to a 1992 study by the Physicians for Responsible Medicine, milk may cause iron deficiencies. Do not take your iron at the same time as caffeine or vitamin E as these will make it less absorbable. Since there are possible side-effects from prolonged ingestion of certain iron supplements, consult with a nutritional expert before adding them to your daily diet.

Food sources: The best sources of iron are liver, oysters, heart and lean meat; leafy greens and molasses are also good sources.

MAGNESIUM

Magnesium is essential for protein synthesis, muscle relaxation, energy production and enzyme production. The intense muscle contractions used in weightlifting and strenuous exercise increase your need for magnesium. The RDA is 350 mg for males and 280 mg for females – but remember, the RDA is always low, and given that so much magnesium is lost in food processing you are receiving much less magnesium from your food than you think.

Recommended dose: 600–1,200 mg daily for athletes. If loose bowels are a problem, adjust the dose accordingly. Note: When calcium and magnesium supplements are taken with iron, your body's ability to absorb iron is impaired.

Food sources: Organic whole grains, dark green vegetables, molasses, nuts, seafood and legumes.

MANGANESE

Manganese is involved in bone and cartilage development, energy production and nerve transmission. It is a catalyst in the synthesis of fatty acids and cholesterol and is part of several important enzymes, including the antioxidant superoxide dismutase. Manganese is essential for the formation of thyroxin, a major constituent of the thyroid gland. A high calcium and phosphorus diet can increase the need for manganese – but very high doses of manganese will result in reduced storage and utilization of iron.

While it is relatively uncommon for North Americans to have high levels of trace manganese in their bodies, a growing body of literature has linked violent behavior to excess manganese. On Groote Eylandt (Island) in Australia (the location of the world's largest manganese mine), the per capita violence and murder rates during a fifty-year period were over 299 percent higher than anywhere else in the country.

The RDA is 2–5 mg daily but because of athletes' high metabolism of glucose and the greater stress placed on their bones and soft tissues, they require more manganese. Most North Americans do not have much manganese in their diets because they eat so much refined food, meat and dairy products.

Recommended dose: 5 mg daily.

Food sources: Whole grains, green leafy vegetables, legumes, pineapples, egg yolks, nuts and black tea.

SILICA

The body transforms the trace mineral silica (silicon dioxide) to a usable form of calcium. Silica is important for bone calcification, the formation of articular cartilage, collagen and connective tissues, and it retards the aging process. Food processing destroys silica.

Recommended dose: 10–25 mg daily.

Food sources: Brown rice, beets, horsetail grass, bell peppers, green leafy vegetables, whole grains and soybeans.

ZINC

Zinc is required by males to normalize testosterone production and maintain healthy reproductive organs. It is also necessary for healthy skin and hair growth and is part of many essential enzymes. Zinc is common in organic foods but it is lacking in commercial products due to food processing and the heavy chemical fertilization of soils. Adolescent males have a greater need for zinc because of their developing reproductive systems. White spots on your finger nails indicate zinc deficiency. Zinc deficiency is common in marathon runners, triathletes, wrestlers and gymnasts. Please note that zinc can interfere with copper assimilation.

Recommended dose: 20–30 mg daily of zinc chelate or zinc gluconate.

Food sources: Sea vegetables, pumpkin seeds, brewer's yeast, garlic, mushrooms, soybeans, oysters and eggs.

ELECTROLYTES: SOMETIMES WATER ISN'T ENOUGH!

True to their name, electrolytes are essential minerals (such as sodium, potassium and chloride) which carry electrical currents throughout the body. Electrolytes control the secretion of hormones and they regulate the osmosis of water between body compartments.

In general, you do not need to supplement your diet with these minerals. An exception may be if you are participating in Ironman distance races or other endurance events lasting three or more hours.

Due to the overabundance of sodium in the North American diet, you are not likely to have a sodium deficiency unless you are taking particular medications. Consumption of alcohol, sugar and coffee, however, will increase the loss of potassium through urination. Do not take additional sodium (salt pills) and limit your general salt intake through foods.

POTASSIUM

Potassium controls the activity of the heart muscles, nervous system and kidneys. If you have poor reflexes, nervous disorders, constipation, irregular pulse or insomnia, have your serum potassium levels checked.

A sodium-potassium balance must be maintained for good health so be careful: excessive intake of salt depletes the body of potassium. Potassium is also lost through urination, sweating and diarrhea, so you should limit or eliminate diuretics (alcohol, sugar and coffee) from your diet. Hypoglycemia affects many athletes and can cause additional potassium loss while sodium and chloride are left in the tissues. In this case, potassium supplements may be required.

Recommended dose: 100–500 mg daily.

Food sources: Avocados, lima beans, potatoes, tomatoes, bananas, fish, dried apricots, spinach and chicken. Food processing upsets the potassium-sodium balance since it adds so much sodium. For example, fresh tuna is 100 parts potassium to 20 parts sodium while canned tuna is 100 parts potassium to 200 parts sodium.

Chloride is part of the salt molecule and if you minimize salt intake you also control chloride levels. Chloride deficiency, just like sodium deficiency, is rarely a problem.

As you can see, virtually any active or sedentary person can benefit from some supplement. I feel that basic nutritional supplements are necessary particularly if your diet contains many refined non-foods, meats and dairy products. Even if you eat a healthy diet based on good foods, I feel that you are still susceptible to deficiencies as a result of nutrient-depleted soils, poor harvesting and storage techniques, food processing and preparation.

Consult with a naturopathic doctor or holistically oriented MD before taking supplements. A professional can test you objectively and then recommend the proper dose and the duration of your supplement program. They should also inform you about the synergistic nature of certain supplements.

We never said looking after yourself would be easy. But, once you learn the ABCs it becomes just another part of your lifestyle.

Chapter 12

Monitoring Your Progress

Just as you should regularly service your car to ensure it is in good running condition, so you should monitor your state of well-being. Unfortunately, too many of us wait for a serious illness before we respond. How often have you seen someone almost get their death certificate before they make a 180-degree turn in their lifestyle?

One of the underlying premises of this book is that an ounce of prevention is worth a pound of cure. If you listen to your body you not only maximize the efficiency of your training, but you can also correct any problems or issues before they get out of hand. By measuring your level of fitness and health quantitatively, you can determine whether you are improving, getting worse or simply plateauing.

· If you listen to your body you will not only maximize the efficiency of your training, but you can also correct any problems before they get out of hand.

· Once you have established your maximum heart rate, you can easily tell if you are performing above or below your optimum level.

· Gradual self-discovery enables you to be more in tune with your body and mind, thus enabling you to improve your training program.

Most good training logs provide plenty of room for you to record your morning heart rate, feelings and eating habits. We do not advocate recording your heart rate, your pH level or nutritional habits every day. Rather, as your health and fitness come into balance you will find that a simple meditation or body check can give you plenty of useful information. It is only when you are starting out or when you realize that your health and fitness levels are out of balance that you will want to closely monitor yourself. You will be amazed how often objective tests will confirm your subjective assessments; soon you will be able to implicitly trust your own instincts.

Many people become committed to their training programs without considering whether the program they are on is right for them. One way to determine this is to have your physical fitness and aerobic capacity tested. Unless you know you are in very good health, you should have a qualified fitness instructor test you. Many fitness clubs, universities and colleges, as well as private fitness institutions, can provide such information for nominal fees. If you are close to a university ask if they are looking for any volunteers for this type of testing. This is how I was first introduced to scientific training and I have never looked back.

Two simple tools you can use to measure your progress are the heart-rate monitor and the pH test. In this chapter we will discuss these and the different ways to calculate target zones to better tailor your workout, the TRIMPS evaluation system, the importance of balancing aerobic and anaerobic exercise and the MAP test for self-monitoring.

HEART-RATE MONITORS

If you experience stress, feel overworked, overindulge in the wrong foods and consume too many spirits, then your body will usually let you know. Our heartbeat is one of the best indicators of how healthy we are and athletes consider it essential to know their active and resting heart rates before they begin their training. While today it is common to see both professional and amateur athletes using heart-rate monitors, back in 1984 when I first started using one, all my friends pointed to the monitor and joked about the precariousness of my health – not to mention my age.

Sally Edwards, a former Ironman winner and author of several triathlon books, was recently quoted in *Triathlete* magazine as saying: "A monitor is much more than just another sports toy that's fun to play with. It's a coach, a training partner and a trusted friend . . . I count on it to never lie about my state of mind or my physical performance."

When starting a training cycle, record your heart rate two to three times a week as soon as you wake up in the morning. This determines your base or resting heart rate. If the pulse rate is more than ten beats per minute higher than your normal resting pulse, it is not a good day to "push." In this case you should consider taking it easy or taking the day off – this way you will reduce the risk of injury and of suppressing your immune system. You should also begin to monitor your eating, sleeping and social habits, and their effect on your body and mind.

For women wearing a bra, a heart-rate monitor chest strap can feel uncomfortable. A simple solution is to sew two pieces of 1.5–2 inch (4 cm) elastic band to the inside of your bra so that the monitor can fit neatly between them. After training simply take the monitor out.

THE PH WONDER!

The pH test can tell you whether you are overtraining or undertraining, whether you are stressed and whether you are eating well. While it may not be as informative as having regular blood work done, the test will tell you if your system is in good health. The test is not just for athletes, but for people with emotional problems such as those who are aggressive, short-tempered or hypersensitive. The pH test is inexpensive, easily done and provides immediate results.

▸ Use a short strip of pH paper and dip it in your urine while urinating. Ideally, do it in the morning to monitor "readiness" and the evening to monitor "stress adaptation."

▸ Take the paper and compare it to the indicator chart provided on the package. The scale usually ranges from 1 (acidic) to 14 (alkaline). Ideally you want to be around 7 (neutral).

▸ If the result is acidic, your system is under stress (check your resting pulse rate – it will likely be slightly elevated).

▸ If the result is too alkaline, then your system likely feels sluggish or, at best, restful.

You can also test the *pH of your saliva* in the morning or evening as mentioned above. In his most recent book, *In Fitness and In Health,* Dr. Maffetone notes that "... oral pH is a good general indicator of fat metabolism. If you need essential fats the pH will be low." Ideally, according to Maffetone, oral pH should read alkaline. Besides, he reports that a high oral pH also protects against cavities.

ACID-ALKALINE METABOLIC BALANCING

This is a very important aspect of health for everyone but it is critical for athletes. Metabolic balancing pertains to the acid-alkaline balance in the body. The alkaline (anabolic) state is the phase where the body rests and restores itself. The acidic (catabolic) state is the phase wherein the body breaks down and expends energy. Ideally, these phases move in cycles: we are alkaline in the morning, becoming more acidic during the day, and then we shift back to a more alkaline state again late in the afternoon.

Most people today are too acidic due to stress and overconsumption of acidic foods. As noted earlier, athletic activity tends to acidify the body and if your pH is too acidic before starting exercise, you could be overstressing your body and be headed for trouble. Make sure you take alkalizing foods after exercise, and on a very regular basis, if your pH is on the acidic side (less than 6.5).

The next best alternative to measuring your blood pH is to check urinary pH. Purchase pH paper from your local drug store and for four or five days check the urine pH at each urination. Put a pH strip in your urine stream and check the color against the color code. A healthy reading is 6.5 during the day and 7.5 in the evening and night. If you are too acid or alkaline, adjust your diet, using Table 12.1. If your pH levels are so acidic that you cannot reduce your acidity merely by eating more alkaline foods, you should try taking greens, barley or chlorophyll powders, and add more seaweed to your diet. It may take a few weeks to two months to normalize your pH level if your diet has been very acidic and if you have been under a lot of stress.

Any long-term deviation from the ideal pH creates illness. Some of the diseases resulting from overacidity are arthritis, cancer, diabetes, migraines and lupus. Excess alkalinity results in diseases such as osteoarthritis as well as constipation, heart problems, bacterial and viral infections and indigestion. If your urine pH is consistently very acidic, have a look at the type of protein and the food combinations you are consuming and follow the tips for optimal protein use (see Chapter 9) which will help reduce acidity. Additional ways to compensate for excess acidity or alkalinity are shown below.

REDUCING EXCESS ACIDITY

If the pH test strip is too yellow, your body is too acidic. Use one or two of the following to help alkalize your body.

► Take a cool bath or shower.

► Have a herbal tea such as peppermint, chamomile, red clover or fenugreek.

- ▸ Drink some fresh vegetable or fruit juice such as pineapple juice or lemon juice with water.

- ▸ Practice deep breathing.

- ▸ If you have tried all of the above methods and are still too acidic, try drinking a mixture of 1/2 tsp (2.5 g) baking soda, 1/4 tsp (1.25 g) cream of tartar, 4 oz (120 ml) water and the juice of one lemon.

REDUCING EXCESS ALKALINITY

Your system is too alkaline if the pH test strip is green or blue. Use one or two of the following techniques to help acidify the body.

- ▸ Have a hot bath or shower.

- ▸ Take 1 tsp (5 ml) vinegar with 1/2 tsp (2.5 g) sea salt in 8 oz (240 ml) water.

- ▸ Drink herbal teas such as raspberry leaf, spearmint and horsetail.

- ▸ Eat low-stress proteins such as soaked seeds, sprouts and tahini (sesame butter).

- ▸ Eat sour pickles, olives or sauerkraut.

Table 12.1 ACIDIFYING AND ALKALIZING FOODS

Please note that this chart refers to how these *foods and vitamins affect the urine pH* not the blood pH.

FOODS	ACIDIFYING	ALKALIZING
Protein:	fish chicken red meat nuts, seeds hard cheeses	soy products eggs almonds milk, yogurt soft cheeses beans
Grains:	whole grains brown rice corn oats barley	refined flour millet
Fruits:	cranberries pomegranates tomatoes	fresh and dried fruits fruit juice
Vegetables:		leafy greens
Miscellaneous:	vinegar unsaturated oils garlic cinnamon horseradish	honey molasses soy sauce pollen seaweed (dulse, nori, kelp)
Vitamins:	B_{12}, B_6 vitamin A beta-carotene vitamin D coenzyme Q_{10}	all other B vitamins vitamin E vitamin K bioflavonoids green drinks

TECHNIQUES FOR CALCULATING YOUR HEART RATE TARGET ZONES

Assuming that you are in good health and are relatively fit, you need to know your maximum heart rate in order to properly tailor your workouts. Once you have established your maximum heart rate, you can easily tell if you are performing above or below your optimum level.

Training, or physical effort, is measured in terms of your heart rate. The aerobic zone (the range in which your aerobic muscles are used to perform an activity) generally ranges from sixty percent to seventy-five percent of your maximum heart rate. When you exceed this level of exertion, your body will begin to use anaerobic muscle, as the aerobic muscle is not able to provide the quick energy needed for intense activity.

Use your maximum heart rate to gauge the intensity of your training.

► Easy workouts should be between 60–70% of your maximal heart rate.

► Endurance workouts between 70–85%.

► Intense workouts at 85% plus.

Four different maximum heart rate calculations are given below. Choose the method which best suits your needs. Dr. Karvonen's formula is the simplest. Dr. Maffetone's formula is excellent for those who are interested in maintaining general fitness and health while Dr. Léger's formula is considered more appropriate for the competitive athlete who is likely to monitor his or her heart rate during each specific workout. Dr. Janssen's formula is perhaps best suited for those who are very sincere and meticulous about their performance level and truly want to fine-tune their efforts. Personally, I subscribe to Léger's formula because over the years I have become more interested in balancing my training with the potential health benefits.

Any of these methods will allow you to objectively and safely monitor your effort and progress. Regardless of the formula you use you might want to consider using a heart-rate monitor to ensure you are neither over- or undertraining. With time you will develop a sense of pace but you still might want to use your heart-rate monitor.

KARVONEN'S TRAINING HEART RATE CALCULATION

Dr. Karvonen has successfully coached numerous world-class athletes to attain world records. To use Dr. Karvonen's training heart rate calculation, you first need to determine your theoretical maximum heart rate.

▸ Theoretical Maximum Heart Rate (T)

    Women: T = 226 minus your age

    Men: T = 220 minus your age

Once you have calculated your theoretical maximum heart rate, apply it to the following formula to calculate your minimum and maximum heart rate.

T = Theoretical Maximum Heart Rate

R = Resting Heart Rate

MIN = (T − R) × .60 + R = Minimum training heart rate

MAX = (T − R) × .85 + R = Maximum training heart rate

You will note that these two figures represent a broad range of exercise effort. Therefore if you are starting out, err on the side of caution. The simplest way to find your starting rate is to find the number that's halfway between your maximum and minimum training heart rates. Stay below the mid-point for aerobic effort and above for anaerobic.

As with all the formulas, pay close attention to your body's response. If you feel faint or dizzy, or you get a side stitch, then slow down or stop. Remember where you are in your training cycle and proceed with caution.

JANSSEN'S HEART RATE CALCULATION

Dr. Peter Janssen, author of *Training, Lactate, Pulse Rate*, who has coached a number of world-class athletes and worked with one of the strongest professional cycling teams from Holland, offers the following technique for measuring maximal heart rate.

1. Be sure you are fully rested and make sure you're healthy enough to undertake a strenuous physical test.

2. Warm up for approximately fifteen minutes so that you feel loose and strong and you are sweating lightly.

3. Do an all-out five-minute run or cycle and for the last thirty seconds really push it. Unless you are really going all out, the procedure will not be very accurate.

4. Your maximum heart rate will then appear on your heart-rate monitor or can be taken from your neck or wrist (although this is less reliable).

   You should also note that a high-impact activity such as running will give a slightly higher maximum heart rate than a low-impact activity.

   Most laboratory tests work on a similar principle, but they usually cost money and are often difficult access. Janssen's test can be done either on your own or with a friend who can encourage you.

LÉGER'S HEART RATE CALCULATION

Another interesting formula recently developed by Dr. Luc Léger, an exercise physiologist at the University of Montréal, takes into consideration a person's age and the type of exercise they are doing. Cycling, for example, will produce a lower heart rate than will running. Léger offers the following formula which will determine your aerobic limits for different sports and enable you to train more efficiently and safely. The following calculations are based on someone who is 38 years of age (see Table 12.2).

HRmax = maximum heart rate

$209 - (age \times .6) = HRmax$ for running
$205 - (age \times .7) = HRmax$ for cycling

Therefore, for a 38 year old, the maximum heart rate for *run-*

ning would be:

HRmax = 209 – [38 × (.6)] = 209 – 22.8 = 186

For the same 38 year old, *cycling*, the maximum heart rate would be:

HRmax = 205 – [38 × (.7)] = 205 – 26.6 = 178

The aerobic zone would be 60–75% of the upper limit, or 107–133 b.p.m.

Table 12.2 HEART RATES FOR SWIMMING, CYCLING AND RUNNING

AGE	UPPER LIMIT HEART RATE		AEROBIC ZONE (60–75%)	
	Swim/Cycle	Run	Swim/Cycle	Run
20	191	197	115–143	118–147
25	188	194	113–141	116–145
30	184	194	111–138	115–143
35	180	188	108–135	113–138
40	177	185	106–133	111–139
50	170	179	102–127	107–134
60	163	173	98–122	104–130

MAFFETONE'S HEART RATE CALCULATION

This formula is from Dr. Philip Maffetone's book *In Fitness and in Health*. Dr. Maffetone practiced applied kinesiology for twenty years and has worked with athletes such as marathoner Grete Waitz and triathlete Mark Allen, among others. His formula is simple:

180 minus your age = your maximum ideal heart rate

► if you have been sick or are presently sick, subtract 10 from your maximum ideal heart rate

► if you have been exercising more than two years, add 5 to your maximum ideal heart rate

For example, if you are 40, and have been training for more

than two years: (180–40) + 5 = 145. Therefore, 145 beats per minute will be your maximum aerobic level before becoming anaerobic.

TRIMPS — TAKING THE GAMBLE OUT OF YOUR TRAINING

Since most of us do not have the time or resources to have our workouts professionally monitored, you can use TRIMPS to accurately measure your exercise and provide you with objective feedback.

Developed by Canadian researcher Dr. Eric Banister, TRIMPS (training impulse score) measures your effort and fatigue in a given activity in order to determine your overall fitness. Of course, we all know that effort is affected by one's level of fatigue (i.e., lack of energy to perform at one's full potential), but most people do not know how to properly balance these elements to maximize the results of their training and reduce the risk of overtraining, plateauing and even injury. It is important, then, to know when it is time to rest and when you can push a little harder.

I believe TRIMPS to be an essential tool for monitoring your progress because it allows you to accurately quantify what you are doing in each of the stages of your training cycle. For example, if you are in your peak phase you will want to do intense workouts over a short period as such intense exercise will give you a higher TRIMPS score. On the other hand, if you are recovering from or tapering for a race, you want to reduce your TRIMPS score so that your body's energy levels can be renewed. By using TRIMPS, then, you can adjust the intensity of your training in a more scientific way and get more out of your training program.

Let us look at how you can use this system to monitor your workouts. Your aim should be to increase your TRIMPS score by ten percent per week. It is best if you can use a heart-rate monitor when applying the TRIMPS method. You will need to calculate the following:

- HRrest: Accurately calculate your resting heart rate. Take your pulse five minutes after waking each morning for five mornings and find the average – assuming you are not suffering from some ailment (e.g., cold, flu or else recovering from an injury).

- HRmax: Calculate your maximum heart rate. You can use any of the formulae explained here or if you prefer, you can do a running calculation. After warming up, run 800 meters as hard as you can, then jog for one minute, then run another all-out 800 meters and measure your heart rate immediately after.

- HRex: As you work out, keep track of how much time you train and what your average heart rate is. Without a heart-rate monitor this can be a bit of a challenge. Several sophisticated heart-rate monitors are available which can calculate your average heart rate (HRex).

Now take these measurements and apply them to the following equation:

$$\text{Training Impulse Score} = \frac{\text{Duration of training} \times (\text{HRex} - \text{HRrest})}{(\text{HRmax} - \text{HRrest})}$$

The following is an example of a TRIMPS score based on a 4-minute swim:

1. HRrest: 60
2. HRmax: 200
3. Duration: 4 minutes
4. HRex: 144
5. $\text{TRIMPS} = \dfrac{4 \times (144 - 60)}{(200 - 60)} = \dfrac{4 \times 84}{140} = \dfrac{336}{140} = 2.4$

Therefore, for your 4-minute swim you collected 2.4 TRIMPS.

You can see that if your HRex was to be 172, and the duration of training was 3 minutes, you would still earn 2.4 TRIMPS!

Quality over quantity – less endurance but greater intensity.

According to Banister, this model can be adapted to any activity, even strength and endurance training. In this case you would need to know:

TRIMPS = number of lifts/reps × percent of maximum lift

1. Calculate your maximum lift for a particular routine (e.g., leg press, bench press, etc.). This figure will be the maximum amount of weight you can lift *once*.

2. Note how many lifts you do per exercise (e.g., 6 lifts/reps per routine).

3. What percentage of your total lift are you lifting? If you lifted 80 kg repeats when your maximum is 100 kg, then it would be 80%.

4. Apply these figures to the formula.

Many athletes I know do not record their strength training as part of their program because they don't know about TRIMPS nor do they consider weights part of a workout because it is not a triathlon event. As was discussed in Chapter 8, however, strength and endurance training *should* be viewed as an essential element of your total fitness and health program.

Using TRIMPS, you can give your workouts real numbers and quantifiable meaning instead of simply recording time or distance. Then using the principle of ten percent increase per week, you can use the scores to guide your improvement on a day-to-day, week-to-week, or even season-to-season basis.

In the April 1995 issue of *Runner's World*, Owen Anderson concludes his review of Dr. Banister's system by saying, "Overall, the Banister system can help you keep a more accurate record of your training. You can then consult this record to analyze your best races and plan for future improvement."

KEEPING A TRAINING LOG

Some training manuals suggest you rate your workouts in terms of intensity and effort. This is fine but often too subjective for practical use. By keeping a daily log you monitor your emotional state, weight, weather conditions, etc. Then by reviewing the information at regular intervals you can assess what your ideal weight and training or racing conditions are. You can also see how long it takes for you to recover and whether you perform better in the morning or at some other time of the day. I have found, however, that once I got to know my performance idiosyncrasies, I could do without the extensive log details. Again, this is an example of gradual self-discovery enabling me to be more in tune with my body and mind, and thereby develop an excellent personal training program. Other than looking impressive, training logs serve minimal purpose for me today. During my Ironman days, I relied almost exclusively on my TRIMPs calculations to guide my workout routines.

By recording how your body responds to different types of workouts, you can tailor your own program to allow for better management of time and effort.

CRITERION PERFORMANCES

Since it is often difficult to quantify skill, emotion and physical capability, you can use a more concrete feedback mechanism to determine your level of progress. You can do this with regular criterion performances. For a triathlete, this might involve doing one performance test per week for three weeks alternating the activity (swim, cycle, run). Thus, in the first week you might be doing a timed 1,000-meter swim in the pool and the following week a 5–10 km run, followed by a 20–30 km time trial on your bike the third week. You then record these performances on a chart or graph to see whether your times improve or not. If they do improve, great; if not, then perhaps you need to assess your training log regarding your feelings, weight, work load, etc. Remember there is no magic formula. You have to constantly monitor your progress. You could also choose one activity and do it every two or three weeks, so long as you compare recent results with previous ones.

YEARLY TRAINING VOLUME – HOW MUCH?

One of the questions we are often asked is: "Is there an ideal volume of training for peak performance whether I am training for a short or a long course?" If there were such a formula, I am sure a lot more people would perform at their top level when called upon to do so. Yet, one need only look at the Olympians or any other top athletes to see that they do not always manage to put it together when needed. Why does this happen?

Developing your own program and monitoring your progress and performance is as much an art form as it is a science. Unfortunately, many athletes have had coaches who have tended to use the same program for everyone without considering how individual differences or external conditions affect athletic ability. While there is generally nothing wrong with generic programs, people are individual and this should be recognized in both work and play if you want the most out of your activities and yourself.

Only recently have we seen a trend whereby athletes and coaches are turning to scientific findings, heart-rate monitors, blood lactate analyses, and nutrition programs to fine-tune their training and racing programs. For over a decade, I have relied on the knowledge of naturopaths to measure my nutritional needs and requirement for supplements. Armed with qualitative and quantitative feedback, you can accurately monitor and develop your own program and take pride in your accomplishments. The science of training and racing has, however, led to other problems such as drug stimulants, blood doping and steroid use. These issues will be addressed in Chapter 14.

Although most of us do not have access to, let alone can afford, a coach, we can still follow the basic advice of many experts and use the *ten percent a year rule*. Many coaches and books recommend increasing your yearly training volume by no more than ten percent per year. However, like Sleamaker, Browning and Banister, we recommend you modify this simple formula somewhat to reflect the "real you." We all know that everyone is different: we have different motivations, various skills and depending on lifestyle and commitments, we have differences in the amount of time we can devote to training. Nevertheless, your motivation, skill and available time can be translated into a quantifiable formula which can be used as a guideline for determining your annual training and racing volume.

ASSESSING YOUR FITNESS LEVEL AND TRAINING VOLUME

1. Assess your basic level of fitness – refer to the tests in the Appendix.

2. Calculate the total number of hours you spent training and racing last year.

3. Assess how good you felt about your year.

4. Using fitness test number 4 (Appendix), and your response to item 3, decide whether you need to do more!

DETERMINE YOUR MAP – MAXIMUM AEROBIC PACE

Once you have developed a solid aerobic base you can perform a simple test to determine whether you are improving your health and fitness or overdoing it.

1. Select a measured distance in swimming, cycling, running or

all three, then measure your level of improvement by testing yourself at the same heart rate over the same distance at equal monthly intervals. Record the length of time it takes to do the same distance at the same heart rate.

2. If your aerobic limit is 140 and it takes you twelve minutes to cover a mile running at this rate, and after a month of training it only takes you eleven minutes at the same heart rate, then you have improved.

3. If, however, it takes you more time to cover the same distance then you are either overtraining or perhaps you have reached your limit. It may be time to introduce some changes to your program or simply accept the fact that age is becoming your great equalizer.

While several researchers have attempted to calculate the aging "handicap," the simple MAP test can determine whether age is catching up with you. The key is training within your aerobic range for seventy-five to eighty-five percent of your workout time. Maffetone and elite athletes such as six-time Ironman winner Mark Allen who use the MAP program, have shown that "proper" training at these levels will result in improved race times.

I advocate basing all your workouts on time as opposed to distance, as this provides a more reliable constant. Your effort can vary dramatically depending on whether you are training at sea level or at 8,000 feet or whether you are running into the wind or with it. If you are following your prescribed heart rate target range for the workout, the prescribed benefits will be the same. Hence, you will be able to stick to your TRIMPs program.

Chapter 13

Treating Injuries Naturally

This chapter looks at the common causes and types of injury, and then gives you information on how to get natural relief through herbal, nutritional and homeopathic means. In addition, I will introduce you to methods of releasing energy that can get blocked throughout your body.

- You can forestall injuries by training properly, balancing fitness and health, and by being mentally prepared for any event.

- If you have an inflammatory condition, you can use a number of foods and supplements to facilitate recovery.

- Proper breathing can make your body less acidic thereby reducing the risk of getting a stress-related illness.

Injuries seem to be an inevitable part of athletics. Some doctors even suggest that injuries are really little more than outward manifestations of our own anxieties and fears. For example, students are notorious for getting sick before exams. First-time marathon runners and Ironman competitors often develop injuries just before or shortly after a race. What this suggests is that certain people will be more prone to injury than others and the causes of their injuries can be explained, in part, by a disharmony between the mind and body. In order to treat sports injuries holistically, then, you need to look at your injuries in a new light.

First, you need to discover the internal conflicts that prevent your body from being in harmony with your emotions. If you are prone to injury or illness then ask yourself: What am I hiding from? What am I trying to avoid? What does the illness or injury really represent for me? Such self-examination requires great inner strength but the rewards are self-discovery – and this will be your biggest aid in the healing process.

While we don't deny that physical injuries do happen (and we have had our share), we would like to encourage you to forestall injuries by training properly, balancing fitness and health, and being mentally prepared for any athletic event.

As many alternative health practitioners have noted, however, few of us are so disciplined that we will not at some time put ourselves at risk of injury. For example, in spite of all the things we know are "wrong" or unhealthy (e.g., speeding, eating junk food, drinking alcohol, smoking and overtraining), we often do many of these things.

INJURIES AND YOUR EMOTIONS

Louise Hay, author of *You Can Heal Your Life*, suggests that we bring on most injuries and ailments by ourselves and that they can often be dealt with through positive thought. In the following chart, Hay suggests possible emotional causes for common problems experienced by athletes.

COMMON PROBLEMS AND PROBABLE CAUSES

PROBLEM	PROBABLE CAUSE
Anxiety	not trusting the flow and process of life
Lower back pain	financial issues
Middle back pain	guilt
Upper back pain	lack of emotional support
Colds	too much going on at once
Fatigue	lack of love for what one does
Injuries (in general)	anger at self, feeling guilty
Knee pain	stubborn ego and pride, inflexibility
Upper leg pain	holding on to childhood traumas
Lower leg pain	fear of the future, not wanting to move

OVERTRAINING

Progressive training continually challenges the body by increasing the intensity, duration and frequency of exercise. This becomes the stimulus for adaptation. Overtraining is when your body is no longer able to adapt because you have allowed too little time for rest and regeneration between challenging workouts.

There are two types of overtraining, both of which can lead to injury:

▸ *Sympathetic.* The symptoms include increased resting heart rate, decreased body mass, disturbed sleep, emotional instability, irritability and excessive sweating.

▸ *Parasympathetic.* These symptoms include anemia, low blood pressure, digestive disturbances and increased hypoglycemic responses.

General symptoms of overtraining include decreased performance (a very clear indicator) and a greater incidence of infections. Some first indicators to watch for are chronic fatigue, depression, insomnia, decreased libido and anxiety.

Rest is the most important aspect of optimum performance especially for athletes whose physical demands are so great. Although some athletes still subscribe to the "no pain, no gain" training routine, your body needs time to regenerate and build its energy, and only rest can give this. You will not lose the foundation that you've built over the long term by taking a few rest days. In fact, if you take two consecutive rest days per week you will perform better than if you push yourself every day.

COMMON ATHLETIC INJURIES

Trying to draw up a list of common athletic injuries is difficult because there are so many sports and so many ways of injuring yourself within each sport. We will focus on six injuries that can befall athletes in any sport. Naturally, some sports will pose a higher risk than others. Common sense should tell you if the injury or condition is caused by poor technique, overuse of certain muscles, weak supporting muscles or even remnants of a prior injury. In such cases, reduce the volume and intensity of your workouts and undertake sport-specific strength training and stretching exercises.

1. *Back pain*. This is probably the most common injury known to athletes and non-athletes alike. Fortunately, most of the discomfort we experience is not serious and is caused by overextension, improper training technique or overuse. Stress, fatigue, weak abdominal muscles and the anxieties of daily life can significantly increase lower back pain.

   Several common ways to prevent lower back pain include: abdominal exercises, stretches that involve bringing one or both knees to the chest and by doing hanging sit-ups – exercises that increase your flexibility and relieve the pressure on the disks in the lower back. (See Figure 13.1.)

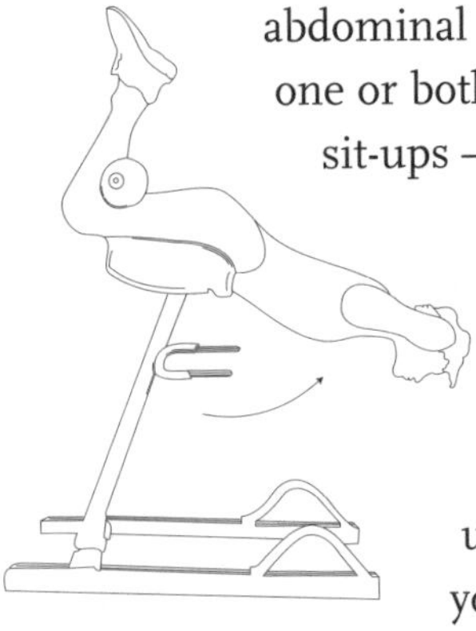

   When doing hanging sit-ups, it is important not to hyperextend your lower back. Inhale as you raise your upper body and exhale as you lower it. If you feel strong, this exercise can be done with weight held against the chest. Be careful to not lift too much weight – go easy. This is but one type of exercise that will help to strengthen your lower back. Consult with a qualified trainer for proper technique.

FIG. 13.1 HANGING SIT-UPS

2. *Knee problems*. Not surprisingly, many knee problems are related to weak lower backs. When the spine does not properly support the body, especially the lower body, any overuse or undue stress in the lower limbs is likely to result in knee problems. Weak or tight quadriceps can also contribute to knee problems.

Knee injuries are among the more common injuries experienced by cyclists, runners, basketball and hockey players. Knee injuries are sometimes referred to as "runner's knee," but true chondromalacia is an irritation of the surface between the kneecap and the cartilage underneath.

Women who overpronate (roll strongly inward on their feet when walking or running) are more likely to get chondromalacia (abnormal softening of the cartilage) than men. Overpronation results in an internal rotation of the knee which can cause the kneecap to track improperly. To avoid these problems, strengthen your back and leg muscles, practice proper technique in your sports and wear appropriate, supportive shoes to prevent knee injuries.

3. *Muscle soreness.* Although muscle soreness is technically not an injury, if you do not pay attention to it, the soreness can develop into an injury. Many inexperienced or weekend athletes overdo an activity and have poor technique. For example, if you haven't played baseball recently but agree to be the weekend pitcher at the family reunion, you might very well end up with sore shoulder muscles.

    Some muscle soreness is normal within forty-eight hours after exercise. It results from increased blood flow in the area where muscle fibers have been broken down. If you have sore muscles you may also experience some swelling, but after a few days of rest or light training, it should go away. In extreme cases of strenuous exertion, such as a marathon, or a mountain hike, the soreness and stiffness will hit you two days after. The Sunday run is felt on Tuesday. The soreness you feel is muscle inflammation and lactic acid setting in.

    You can prevent this by maintaining regular and balanced workouts, but not doing the same thing every day. Work up to your goal. Build strength by *progressively* increasing the duration and intensity of your activities.

4. *Strains and sprains.* These injuries to muscles or connective tissue (tendons, ligaments and fascia), result from both acute trauma (such as twisting your ankle on uneven ground) or chronic overuse (bench pressing more than you are comfortable with). A strain results from a muscle or connective tissue being overworked; a sprain is an actual break or rupture in the tissue and usually causes more intense pain and swelling. Sprains usually take longer to heal than do strains.

5. *Muscle pulls and muscle tears.* As with strains and sprains, acute stress or overuse can result in muscle pulls and tears. In both cases, the muscle is extended beyond its ability to meet the demands placed on it. When this occurs you can either end up with tiny pulls or tears in the muscle fibers or, more seriously, incapacitating the muscle altogether. If sprinters are not properly warmed up and in good physical condition, their explosive power can overload the hamstring leading to a pull or, more seriously, a tear.

   Depending on your sport, the location of pulls and tears will vary: shoulder muscles are the most vulnerable for swimmers, the inner thigh for soccer and hockey players and the calf for aerobic dancers. While pulls and tears can be more debilitating than strains and sprains, they can be avoided if you learn to pay attention to how your body is feeling. Soreness is usually an early warning sign. Once you have a pull or a tear the recovery can take some time. Again, make sure to warm up completely before beginning any exercise.

6. *Tendinitis.* Knowing the difference between tendinitis and a strain is not always easy. Like most of the injuries covered in this section, tendinitis results from overuse. This condition usually occurs in the ankles, feet, knees, shoulders and wrists. Under excessive stress the tendons develop microscopic tears. Sometimes the inflammation, stiffness and pain will subside after the tendon has been warmed up and you work through any lingering discomfort. Consequently,

the injury may persist for a long time and can escalate into something more serious. Even minor inflammations, therefore, should not be taken lightly.

While this list is by no means exhaustive, it does represent some of the more common injuries. Other frequent injuries include bursitis – an inflammation around the bone and cartilage of the major joint being exercised; stress fractures – minute breaks in the bone resulting from excessive use; shin splints – similar to a stress fracture in sensation but usually less serious.

TREATING INFLAMMATORY CONDITIONS

Naturopaths, osteopaths, chiropractors and medical doctors fre-

BASIC FIRST AID

First aid treatment for most sports injuries is summed up by the term RICE – Rest, Ice, Compression and Elevation.

· *Rest.* Avoid all pain-causing activity.

· *Ice.* Wrap an ice pack in a towel and apply to areas where circulation will not be impaired. Ice for twenty minutes to one hour or until the pain and swelling subside. *Usually ice reduces pain, but if it increases it then use a heating pad.* For muscular injuries, apply only heat.

· *Compression.* Sprains swell up as a bodily defense to restrict movement and prevent further damage. Apply tensor bandages to the sprained area and check your blood circulation every thirty minutes to make sure it is flowing throughout the sprain without impediment.

· *Elevation.* Elevate the injured limb if possible.

quently treat patients suffering from strains, sprains and other musculoskeletal injuries. Their treatments range from chiropractic adjustments to physiotherapy and nutrition supplements. The most common treatment in conventional medicine is the use of cortisone, which definitely reduces inflammation but when used repeatedly produces many undesirable side-effects.

The adrenal glands produce cortisone in normal amounts but when external cortisone is supplied, the body decreases its own cortisone production and over the long term this can cause severe adrenal gland dysfunction.

Cortisone is given primarily for the inflammations caused by injury. The inflammatory response, however, is actually one of the body's natural systems of defense. Fibroblasts, members of the body's defense army, are also suppressed when cortisone is given, and this can actually delay healing.

Other symptoms associated with chronic use of cortisone and other steroids are progressive joint deterioration, decreased bone mineral density, electrolyte imbalances, hormonal dysfunctions, gastrointestinal problems and decreased cartilage synthesis when cortisone is injected into joints.

From a naturopathic perspective, there is little place for the continued or frequent use of cortisone for sports injuries. There are many natural alternatives to cortisone therapy for musculoskeletal problems, some of which are discussed below. Remember that the body can incur structural problems from injury or just from training. If structural problems are left untreated, you can experience more serious back or other health problems in the future. I would strongly advise regular visits to a chiropractor or osteopath who is familiar with athletic training and injuries.

HERBAL SUPPORT FOR INFLAMMATORY CONDITIONS

The following list is not exhaustive, rather, it includes some of the readily available and proven herbal support remedies recommended for inflammatory conditions. And while a recommended dose is given, for persistent inflammation always consult a trained practitioner.

▸ *Bupleurum.* This herb contains steroid-like molecules, is a potent anti-inflammatory and an excellent support for the adrenals.

Recommended dose: Bupleurum is usually combined with other Chinese herbs in formulas that support the kidneys and alleviate liver congestion. If you want to use this herb individually for its adaptogenic properties, then I would recommend putting one teaspoon of the root bark in one-half pint of water. Bring the water to a boil and simmer for thirty minutes. Drink two or three cups daily – warm or cold.

> *Curcumin*. This herb has a long history of use in ayurvedic medicine for the treatment of sprains and internal inflammations.

THE CASTOR OIL PACK

This is a standard naturopathic treatment for trauma. Buy a good quality castor oil from your local health food store – not the drug store. In case of injury, apply the oil as follows:

Soak a flannel or wool cloth in the castor oil and apply to the injured area. Cover with a plastic bag then apply heat (a hot water bottle or a heating pad) for twenty to thirty minutes. Do this two or three times daily. This is an old folk remedy that really works.

Recommended dose: 400–600 mg three times daily.
Please note that curcumin is an active component of turmeric however taking turmeric is not the same as taking curcumin – one would have to take approximately 20,000–60,000 mg of turmeric to get the same results.

> *Licorice Root* (Western and Chinese). Glycyrrhizin and other active components in licorice root inhibit prostaglandin synthesis (which causes inflammation). Taking licorice root as an adjunct to cortisone therapy can support the adrenals and can help prevent some of the side-effects of cortisone.

Recommended dose: Two to four 380 mg tablets taken before meals. The deglycyrrhizinated licorice does not cause gastrointestinal upsets. For more information, see the section on adaptogenic herbs in Chapter 14.

> *White Willow Bark*. This remedy is well known for its pain-relieving and anti-inflammatory qualities. For over two thousand years, Chinese physicians have used willow bark to treat

pain and fever in the same way that North Americans use acetylsalicylic acid (ASA) today. Willow bark, however, does not cause the side-effects of ASA.

Recommended dose: 20–40 mg two or three times daily.

NUTRITIONAL SUPPORT FOR INFLAMMATORY CONDITIONS

If you have an inflammatory condition you can use a number of foods and supplements to facilitate recovery. Again, this is not a comprehensive list, but it does include essential and readily available products.

▶ *Bromelain.* Bromelain is a proteolytic enzyme isolated from the pineapple plant. Beneficial results have been obtained by using proteolytic enzymes as anti-inflammatory agents in sports injuries and in some degenerative diseases.

Recommended dose: 1 g twice daily between meals.

▶ *Flavonoids.* Flavonoids are a group of plant pigments which are useful in the treatment of many conditions such as reducing inflammation and stabilizing collagen structures. Currently, one of the most commonly used single flavonoids is proanthocyanidin in the form of grape see or pine bark.

Recommended dose: During the healing process I would recommend 200–300 mg daily. Once the injury is healed you can continue to use flavonoids for their antioxidant effect, though you should decrease the dose to 100–150 mg daily. Flavonoids also come in the form of "mixed flavonoids" offering approximately 20 mg of citrus flavonoids and 400 g of non-citrus flavonoids per capsule. I recommend taking three capsules daily.

▶ *Omega-3 Essential Fatty Acid* (Alpha-linolenic Acid). The value of essential fatty acids is discussed in Chapter 9. Omega-3 is particularly important in the anti-inflammatory process. Eicosapentanenoic acid (EPA), a form of omega-3 fatty acid found in fish oil, can also be taken to alleviate inflammation.

Recommended dose: 1,000 mg three times daily. The fish that contain the highest concentrations of EPA are anchovies, salmon, herring, mackerel and tuna.

▸ *Vitamin A.* In its beta-carotene form, vitamin A has strong antioxidant and anti-inflammatory qualities, and is necessary for collagen synthesis and wound healing.

Recommended dose during healing: 100,000–150,000 IU daily. Avoid during pregnancy.

▸ *Vitamin C.* This vitamin is essential for the prevention and repair of injuries. It forms and maintains collagen which is a component of tendon and bursae tissue.

Recommended dose during healing: Take at bowel tolerance level.

▸ *Vitamin E* and *Selenium.* These are antioxidants which decrease free radicals, an important part of relieving inflammation. Vitamin E generally accelerates healing.

Recommended dose during healing: 1,200–1,600 IU daily.

▸ *Zinc.* This mineral significantly quickens the healing of wounds and is an antioxidant. It also stabilizes membranes, synthesizes collagen and reduces inflammation.

Recommended dose: 30–50 mg daily.

HOMEOPATHY

The homeopathic system of medicine uses remedies made from natural substances (animal, vegetable and mineral), which are manufactured according to strict pharmacological methods, and are safe, non-toxic and have no side-effects. German physician Samuel Hahnemann introduced this system of medicine approximately two hundred years ago although the roots of homeopathy date back to fourth century Greece where Hippocrates was developing his famous philosophy of natural health.

The term homeopathy comes from the Greek *homeo* meaning similar, and *pathos* meaning suffering. Homeopathy is based on the law of similars which means like cures like. This law of similars states that a substance, which causes symptoms of illness in a healthy person, when specially prepared and taken in diluted amounts, will cure a sick person who has the same symptoms.

The fundamental principles upon which homeopathy is based are:

► The body has an innate capacity to heal itself and to re-establish balance.

► Homeopathic remedies are given to enhance the body's own abilities to heal itself.

► A person who is ill or injured is treated according to the specific symptoms displayed.

► It is the person who is treated, not the disease.

► Treatment takes into account mental and emotional symptoms as well as physical symptoms.

HOW DO I USE HOMEOPATHIC REMEDIES?

For small aches and pains, minor injuries from sports or other traumas, you can use homeopathic remedies. For the more chronic complaints, you should consult with a naturopathic physician, a homeopath, or a holistic practitioner trained in homeopathy.

Use the symptoms listed below to help you choose the correct remedy. In general, take lower potencies (anything under 30c) of the remedy every half hour until improvement is noted. Treatment should stop when there are signs of improvement. If there is a relapse, take the indicated remedy again. Remedies are taken under the tongue and held for approximately thirty seconds.

Homeopathics should be taken at least twenty minutes before or after you have eaten, and the further away from food the better. Some substances like coffee, peppermint, toothpaste, essential oils or camphor can neutralize the activity of the homeopathic remedy. You can, however, take these remedies with water.

I have mentioned the most common remedies to use in various circumstances. You can apply the remedies to *any* injury that has the indicated symptoms, regardless of location on the body.

HOMEOPATHIC REMEDIES FOR PHYSICAL INJURIES — STAGE ONE

Consider using one of these remedies in the first twenty-four hours following an injury. Please note the same dose applies to each remedy unless otherwise indicated. Take a low potency (under 30c) every fifteen minutes for severe pain then take once every four hours as symptoms improve (usually after one to four hours).

▸ *Arnica*. This remedy is the number one homeopathic first aid remedy and it should be considered first for any injury. The basic symptoms to look for are: aches and bruises, dislocations and sprains and soreness after overexertion. If the injury feels better when you lie down, improves with a cold compress or feels worse when you touch it, you should consider using *Arnica*.

Please note, in cases of *injury with shock* use a high-potency *Arnica*, initially (200c) every four hours for twenty-four hours, or until better.

▸ *Bryonia*. This remedy acts on the serous membranes, joints and muscles. *Bryonia* is recommended when you have aching in every muscle or muscle tearing, dryness of the mucous membranes and when you are grumpy. Injuries that feel better when heat and pressure are applied, but feel worse when cooled or in motion, should also be treated with *Bryonia*.

▸ *Bellis perennis*. Use if *Arnica* didn't work in the first one to four hours. *Bellis* acts upon the blood vessels and muscle fibers. This is the first remedy to consider when there is muscle soreness or

injuries to the deeper tissues and nerves. It is an excellent remedy for sprains and strains. If you feel cold and chilly, the injury is
black and blue, and feels better when it is heated or rubbed but
feels worse when ice or cold are applied, *Bellis* is recommended.

When you have an acute injury, you should immediately
consider using *Arnica* or *Bellis*. Decide which one you should
take based on your symptoms (i.e., if you are sore, achy and feeling better with warmth, then use *Arnica*).

► *Homeopathic creams.* These creams, used with or without an
internal remedy, can be applied topically to an injury, unless
you have skin abrasions. *Arnica* is a wonderful remedy and
can be applied at all stages of the healing process.

HOMEOPATHIC REMEDIES FOR PHYSICAL INJURIES — STAGE TWO

If after the first twenty-four hours you have not found relief
from the stage one remedies, try one of the remedies from the
following list. These may be given four times daily until pain
and stiffness are better.

► *Hypericum.* This is the greatest remedy for injuries to the
nerves, especially in the extremities. Consider using
Hypericum to alleviate sharp nerve pain such as when your
fingers are caught in a door or when you injure your tailbone.

► *Phytolacca.* This remedy has a powerful effect on the fibrous
and osseous tissue, fasciae and muscle; it also works particularly well on the Achilles' tendon and ankle joints. Aching,
soreness, restlessness and prostration should be treated with
Phytolacca. If the injury feels better with rest and elevation and
worse when you move, use *Phytolacca.*

► *Rhus tox.* A good remedy for pain in the small of the back and
knee joint. *Rhus tox* affects fibrous tissue, particularly joints

and tendons that are painful and stiff. It is always good to consider *Rhus tox* in cases of sprains and strains, plantar fasciitis
and tendinitis. It is also very good for arthritis. If the injury
improves with continued movement and applications of heat,
Rhus tox is recommended.

▸ *Ruta*. This remedy acts on the cartilage and periosteum. It is
excellent for healing strained flexor tendons and when all
parts of your body feel painful as if bruised. *Ruta* is good for
bruised shins, bursitis, sprains and when your hamstrings feel
shortened. The symptoms indicating *Ruta* are similar to those
for *Rhus tox*, but *Ruta* is recommended when the pain feels
like it is deep in the bone.

CLEANSING WOUNDS

You should not use creams on open wounds. Rather, clean the
wound with hydrogen peroxide or iodine then use a solution of
Calendula oil or tincture diluted in water. Soak a sterile gauze
pad then apply it directly to the wound, covering it with plastic
wrap. Change the dressing every four hours moistening the
gauze before removing, so you don't pull off the scab that is
forming. Leave the wound open at night so the air can help
healing. Use *Calendula* cream or *Symphytum* ointment once the
wound has closed up. The homeopathic remedy *Hepar sulph* is
also beneficial for healing abrasions or scrapes. *Use creams only
when the skin is intact.*

FRACTURES

After taking *Arnica* for initial trauma, the most common remedy for knitting together fractured bones is *Symphytum*, the
homeopathic form of comfrey. Take every two hours until pain
is diminished then four times daily.

SUNSTROKE AND HEAT EXHAUSTION

A muscle cramp may be the first sign of a heat problem, along with nausea, vomiting, dizziness and fainting. Continuing to run while showing these symptoms may lead to a stroke. When the core body temperature rises more than 35°F (2°C), permanent physical and mental changes can occur. Get out of the sun and seek immediate medical attention in cases of heat stroke or exhaustion.

If you think you are suffering from sunstroke or heat exhaustion, you should do the following:

▸ drink water immediately

▸ lie down

▸ cover your body with blankets

▸ call medical staff

▸ take one of the following homeopathic remedies every fifteen minutes: *Arnica, Belladonna* (recommended if you have a hot head, cold feet, dilated pupils and a violent response – these symptoms generally accompany the sudden onset of sunstroke), *Nat carb* (indicated when you are thirsty, nervous and oversensitive to light and noise) or *Glonoin* (for when you have no thirst, a dry mouth, cold extremities, a hot, flushed head and when any exposure to the sun makes you feel worse).

BURNS AND SUNBURNS

Take *Arnica* immediately for shock, then apply a *Calendula* tincture as a dressing over the burn (mix one-half teaspoon of *Calendula* tincture to one cup water) to relieve pain and promote healing. Take the appropriate homeopathic remedy every ten to fifteen minutes as needed.

▸ *Aloe vera.* An excellent healing remedy for all burns. To use, cut a piece of the herb and apply the gel directly to the skin.

▸ *Apis.* Use for first-degree burns if *Urtica* doesn't work.

▸ *Causticum.* Use for second-degree burns accompanied by blistering.

▸ *Cantharis.* Use for third-degree burns or acid burns.

▸ *Urtica urens.* Use for first-degree burns which are accompanied by itching and stinging.

BITES AND STINGS

Use *Apis* where there may be allergic reactions. If your wound feels better with cold and worse with heat, use A*pis. Ledum* is a good remedy for puncture wounds such as dog bites, wasp or bee stings, and when your skin feels better when cold is applied.

HEAD INJURIES

Always consider *Arnica* for a head injury. Other remedies include *Nat sulph* for chronic headaches that have plagued you since an injury and which are accompanied by personality change or depression. Consider *Hypericum* for sharp shooting pains and nerve damage.

RELEASING BLOCKED ENERGY

I would like to introduce some of the more effective ways of releasing blocked energy including acupressure, reflexology, *qi gong* breathing, color breathing, magnetic therapy and several bodywork methods. I consider massage to be a type of energy therapy. Most people think massage is just a technique of working tension and toxic build-up out of the muscles. This is only part of the picture. Massage also affects the body's subtle energies by using the acupuncture points, meridians and the flow of *chi* (energy). Some therapists are very sensitive and can release energy into any part of the body when particular points are worked. These therapies can be an invaluable way to maintain optimum health and performance in all areas of life.

ACUPRESSURE

Acupressure is an ancient method of relieving pain by applying pressure to the skin on certain parts of the body. Just underneath the surface of the skin there is a complex network of meridians which carry *chi* from one part of the body to another. When pressure is applied to a point along a meridian, energy is released and carried to those organs that lie along the same meridian. The points used in acupressure are the same as those used in acupuncture but no needles are used. Stimulating points by pressure, heat or needles releases endorphins which are the neurochemicals that relieve pain. Not only is acupressure an excellent method of relieving stress, joint stiffness, digestive complaints, colds, backache and menstrual discomfort, it also enhances the immune and hormone systems. This is a simple therapy that requires no special equipment and is safe to do on yourself.

QI GONG BREATHING TO BALANCE ENERGY

This is a set of breathing exercises that you may want to try if you wish to improve concentration and build your energy, and at the same time revitalize and relax yourself. The foundation of *qi gong* (pronounced chi-gong) is abdominal breathing – a technique that any athlete can adopt. Most people have never been trained to breathe properly and so only their upper chest rises during athletic or quiet activity. This is unhealthy since shallow breathing makes the body more acidic which, in turn, creates more potential for stress-related illnesses. *Qi gong* also uses visualization techniques to intensify and deepen breath.

Qi gong offers very simple breathing exercises that you can do daily to balance your flow of energy. After awhile the breathing techniques will take less concentration and effort and you will also be able to do them when you are training or racing.

REFLEXOLOGY

Reflexology, like acupressure, is a way to relieve pain in one part of the body by applying pressure to another part of the body – in this case the feet or hands. All internal glands and organs are connected to nerve endings in the hands and feet. By stimulating a certain area on the sole of a foot, for example, you can send an electro-chemical nerve impulse to its corresponding organ, thus stimulating the organ. Everyone from the weekend athlete to the professional relies on good physical and mental abilities to help them play, work well and win. This technique can be used by people of all ages. It is safe, simple and can improve your health in a great many ways. For example, reflexology:

- improves circulation
- increases endurance
- heightens concentration
- rids the body of toxins
- enhances the body's natural healing abilities
- opens and clears blocked energy "highways"
- restores vitality
- reduces stress and tension
- induces relaxation

INCREASE YOUR ENERGY BY BREATHING COLOR

This is a visualization technique you can use to attain a variety of mental states. As each color affects your psyche differently, you can put yourself into different states of mind by using the simple meditation technique described below. It is well known that the eye can register color oscillations and that color can affect the psyche. All light is visible energy that travels in waves, and each color has a different wavelength. To see if you can feel any effects of color try this experiment.

All you need to do is to sit or lie down, close your eyes and imagine a vivid hue of a color. Once you start seeing this color then visualize yourself breathing this color into your lungs. (You should incorporate *qi gong* breathing into this exercise.) Breathe deeply three times. Then imagine this color flowing through your whole body. Repeat this breath three times. Then take another deep breath, and this time picture the color flowing throughout your whole body. Red is associated with power, energy, vitality and excitement of life. Breathing red can stimulate strength, joy, happiness and love. Blue is the color of peace and relaxation. It is often used to treat pain and congestion. Yellow promotes digestion, stimulates the muscles and stabilizes the nerves. Green promotes feelings of contentment and tranquility. It increases vitality, supports overall health and can decrease joint inflammation. Orange increases one's sense of ambition and enthusiasm. It is also considered helpful for cramps and spasms and is very powerful for the thyroid.

MAGNETIC THERAPY

This therapy, which dates back to the ancient Egyptians, uses magnetic fields to provide relief from pain and to prevent disease. Pulsing or static magnets are used to influence the electromagnetic impulses sent by the brain to other parts of the body and can be used to interrupt the transmission of pain signals. With magnetic therapy, knee braces can be removed more quickly, weightlifters can reduce lower back pain and sciatica, and carpal tunnel syndrome can be relieved. Magnetic therapy can halve the normal healing time for muscle, tendon and soft tissue injuries. Furthermore, it reduces the need for medications. Headaches, arthritis, back pain, tension and blood pressure disorders can all be treated with magnetic therapy. It has no known unwanted long-term side-effects.

AN OVERVIEW OF BODYWORK TECHNIQUES

Bodywork aims to enhance health and improve body structure and functions through various techniques such as massage, deep breathing exercises and manipulation of the body and its energy fields. Many different types of bodywork exist. Many bodywork practitioners, including chiropractors and massage therapists, use a combination of techniques.

The following is a general overview of bodywork techniques and therapies.

▸ *Alexander Technique.* A combination of massage and manipulation which focuses on alleviating the tension that results from bad posture and movement patterns. The Alexander technique has helped athletes improve performance and relieve chronic pain.

▸ *Craniosacral Therapy.* I find this therapy very powerful. It is based on the concept that the bones in your skull are constantly moving within the cerebrospinal fluids thus causing your head to expand and contract. Gentle manipulation of your skull will move the cerebrospinal fluid around the spine and down into the sacrum. This subtle movement results in the realignment of your bones so that they resume their natural position and function.

▸ *Feldenkrais.* Based on the premise that the body is a mirror of the mind, Feldenkrais focuses on improving your awareness of unconscious movements, stance and body patterns. The benefits are increased vitality and overall well-being. The Feldenkrais method is useful for people, such as athletes, who need to improve their performance and it is also excellent for those whose movements are limited by pain or disability.

- *Reiki.* Through touch and gentle brushing of the "energetic" field, the natural energy flow is restored which enables the body to heal itself at the emotional, mental, spiritual and physical levels.

- *Rolfing®.* Also known as structural integration. This deep connective tissue massage is designed to realign your body and improve posture. Research indicates that this technique promotes more energetic and smoother body movements.

- *Shiatsu*: Like acupressure, shiatsu involves applying pressure along your body's energy meridians to stimulate *chi,* your intrinsic life force.

- *Therapeutic Touch®.* Involves the transfer of energy through touch or by holding the hands over various parts of your body. Scientific studies have shown that this technique can increase the oxygen carrying capacity of red blood cells and can effectively treat musculoskeletal problems.

- *Trager.* This is a method of alleviating back pain, emotional trauma and musculoskeletal problems by gently manipulating the muscles and joints. Many athletes find that this therapy makes their movements more efficient and increases their stamina.

When all is said and done, self-knowledge, a good diet and proper preparation are the best ways to ward off injury. Those athletes who put themselves through rigorous training often must contend with a different sort of injury – stress. This will be examined in the next chapter, followed by a discussion of the many ergogenics available to enhance your performance.

Chapter 14

Adaptogens and Ergogenics

The adaptation required of the body during vigorous training is one very important facet of sports physiology that is ignored by most athletes and trainers. In this chapter we will tell you how to use natural substances to help your body deal with the added demands of athletics. These will also improve the overall functioning of your body.

The *general adaptation syndrome* was first studied by Hans Seyle and gives us a greater understanding of the body's ability to adapt to stress. Stress is a relative term which we need to define before going any further. In his book *The Stress of Life*, Seyle defined stress as the non-specific response of the body to any demand (pleasurable or unpleasant) made upon it.* The body has to adapt to many different types of stress such as:

· While training, your body is under prolonged stress, and your adrenal glands must constantly adapt to these demands.

· If you want to incorporate exercise into your lifestyle, adrenal assessment will be an important part of your training program.

· Tonic herbs improve the assimilation of nutrients which, in turn, increases the energy and strength of the body.

► *Physical stress.* Allergies, backaches, hypertension, infections, overwork, overtraining, lack of sleep, chronic inflammation, chronic pain or illness and light cycle disruption (usually experienced by shift workers).

*Adapted from *The Stress of Life*, © 1956 by Hans Seyle. New York: McGraw-Hill. Reproduced with the permission of the McGraw-Hill Companies.

▸ *Chemical stress.* Toxic metal exposure, environmental pollution, junk food diets, alcohol, tobacco, caffeine and drugs.

▸ *Thermal stress.* Overheating or overcooling of the body.

▸ *Barometric stress.* Shifts in barometric pressure during major weather changes.

▸ *Emotional and mental stress.* Anger, fear, worry and anxiety.

▸ *Electromagnetic stress.* Personal computers, fluorescent lights, hair dryers, microwave ovens, power lines, televisions and waterbeds.

Throughout the day your body automatically adapts to stress without any obvious symptoms. Nevertheless, the body does need to adapt whether the stress is pleasant or unpleasant. In general, the greater the stress, the more difficult it will be for you to adapt. If you are over-stressed, you will most likely experience the physical symptoms related to adrenal dysfunction. This is because the adrenals are primary organs that respond to stress.

This information is important if you are just beginning to incorporate exercise into your lifestyle and for athletes who train regularly. We all experience various levels of stress in our lives which directly affect the health of the adrenals. Most people are familiar with negative stress-related emotions such as fear and anxiety. Few, however, realize that positive stress such as over-excitement or great anticipation also force the body to adapt.

THE ADRENALS — THE "STRESS" GLANDS

The adrenal glands are critical to our sense of well-being because they are our primary stress adaptation organs. When these glands are overworked, you can become physically or emotionally ill. Unfortunately, the adrenals are largely ignored by conventional medicine. Unless eighty to ninety percent of the organ function is gone (a condition known as Addison's disease), conventional medicine does not recognize the symptoms associated with hypoadrenalism (poor adrenal performance). The loss of function in this gland is called the *adrenal syndrome* and it is epidemic – I see it in athletes and patients of all ages. The athlete, in particular, is under prolonged stress while training or racing, and the adrenals must constantly adapt to these demands.

The adrenal glands are composed of two parts, the medulla (inner portion) and the cortex (outer portion). Stress on the body causes the medulla to increase epinephrine secretion which, in turn, causes the adrenal cortex to produce greater amounts of corticoids, namely cortisol. Cortisol stimulates the formation of new glucose from protein and fat, and decreases the use of glucose by other cells of the body. The result of this chain of action is to provide the energy needed by the body when exercising. Sustained blood sugar levels are very important to the athlete because of the high energy demands placed on the body during exercise. Athletes who strive to reach their optimum potential require an efficient metabolism to manage their high energy requirements.

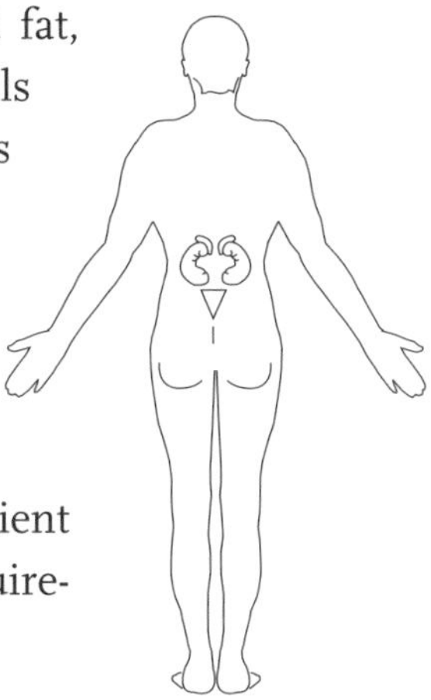

The secretion of cortisol in response to stress is one of the most important functions of the adrenals. If the stress is prolonged, the

FIG. 14.1 LOCATION OF THE ADRENAL GLANDS

adrenals can become fatigued. Many hypoadrenal individuals, especially those who train regularly, can maintain normal serum cortisol levels in a resting state, but they have no adrenal reserve. This means that the adrenal glands of these individuals are working just enough to keep up with normal activities but they lack the reserve to respond to any additional stress. It is common for athletes to participate in a race only to become extremely ill afterwards. They do not have any adrenal reserve to draw on after such intense competition. Fatigued adrenal glands diminish the function of the immune system.

SYMPTOMS OF HYPOADRENALISM

Please keep in mind that you may not experience any symptoms unless you stop training. This is because regular exercise constantly stimulates the adrenals to produce hormones. It is only when your body rests that these symptoms may appear.

MAJOR SYMPTOMS ASSOCIATED WITH ADRENAL DYSFUNCTION

excessive fatigue	low body temperature
nervousness/irritability	hypoglycemia
low back pain	insomnia
cravings for sweets	poor resistance to infection
dry, thin skin	difficulty building muscle
alcohol intolerance	inability to concentrate
light-headedness	light sensitivity
depression	pain and spasm in sternomastoid/ trapezius muscles

As a naturopathic doctor, I look at the early signs of a deficiency in the organs. I would not recommend waiting until you start developing these symptoms before you begin supporting the adrenal glands with nutrients. Should the adrenals become severely exhausted, as in cases of chronic fatigue syndrome or fibromyalgia, it is a long climb back before you can have normal adrenal function.

Other organs commonly associated with poor adrenal function are the pituitary and the thyroid glands. I recommend having an organ status evaluation made by a naturopathic physician or holistic medical doctor if you are presently in training or are about to embark upon an aggressive training cycle. I have seen too many professional and amateur athletes burn out to the point where climbing stairs is an effort. The reason for this usually is poor adrenal function.

If you who are looking to incorporate exercise into your "get healthy" program, adrenal assessment is a very important part of smart training.

SUPPLEMENTS FOR HEALTHY ADRENAL FUNCTION

▸ *Adrenal glandulars.* Glandular preparations facilitate the conversion of appropriate substrates into hormones. Please note that the glandulars *do not* contain steroids themselves and are not the hormone adrenaline. They are derived from animal adrenal glands and when properly processed they contain small but active concentrations of enzymes capable of converting cholesterol to corticosteroids. One of the most important corticosteroids is cortisol which maintains your body's blood sugar balance.

Recommended dose: 100–200 mg two to four times daily as needed.

▸ *Pantothenic Acid.* As stated, the adrenal cortex is designed to respond to stressful situations by secreting steroid hormones which initiate and maintain a variety of physiological reactions. Pantothenic acid is a component of coenzyme A and is crucial to the adrenals' ability to affect fatty acid synthesis, steroid synthesis and carbohydrate and protein metabolism. Pantothenic acid is also responsible for converting choline to acetylcholine which improves endurance, athletic performance and memory.

Recommended dose: 1,000–2,000 mg daily.

▸ *Vitamin C.* The adrenals have the highest concentration of vitamin C of any tissue in the body with the exception of the brain.

Recommended dose: If your adrenals need support, I recommend high doses of ester-C (1,000–3,000 mg) or vitamin C with bioflavonoids (1,000–5,000 mg). The dose will depend on your bowel tolerance. If you experience gas or loose stools then decrease your dose until these symptoms disappear. Vitamin C with bioflavonoids has synergistic effects when taken with pantothenic acid.

In addition to the aforementioned nutrition supplements, there are many sources of adrenal support to be found in the herbal kingdom. These herbs fall into the *adaptogen* and *tonic* categories.

THE AMAZING HERBAL KINGDOM

From ancient times humans have looked to the herbal kingdom for treatments for illness. Remedies were determined through trial and error, watching animals and trusting intuition. The information gathered by our ancestors has been refined over time to the point where today, laboratory techniques are used to standardize the potency of herbal products. Adaptogenic herbs are a prime area of interest in research currently and there are numerous studies validating the effectiveness of botanical medicines.

WHAT ARE ADAPTOGENS?

Adaptogens increase the body's ability to cope with physical, chemical and biological stress. The most important part of stress adaptation is the ability of the body to maintain high tissue energy. When the adrenal glands have great demands placed on them for prolonged periods of time, they become fatigued, and if we keep challenging them it is like whipping a tired horse – the horse picks up and moves on a bit but at some point it will be unable to respond to the whipping and will fall in complete exhaustion. If you continue to drive your body and make exorbitant demands on your adrenals, you will have a greater price to pay down the road than if you had listened to your body, slowed down and allowed yourself to rest.

Adaptogenic substances have many characteristics but the most important is their *normalizing effect regardless of the condi-*

tion of the individual. They are non-toxic and will help your body regain and maintain balance. Among the many beneficial effects of using adaptogens are:

- improved glucose tolerance
- decreased stress
- increased stamina and endurance
- protection and support of your immune system
- increased protein synthesis
- strengthened cardiovascular and respiratory systems
- better ability to adapt in situations of extreme heat, cold, altitude and pressure.

I cannot overemphasize the importance of incorporating adaptogenic substances into your exercise support program.

ADAPTOGENIC HERBS FOR THE ATHLETE

- Astragalus *(Astragalus membranaceus)*. This is an adaptogen highly recommended for younger athletes. It is superior to ginseng and has the advantage of being much cheaper. It strengthens the arms and legs and energizes the whole body. Some experts recommend that young people use astragalus as it affects their "physical energy" more, and that older people use ginseng as it affects the "mental energy" more.

   Athletes of all ages can blend either a good quality Panax ginseng or Siberian ginseng with astragalus and licorice. This will affect the inner and outer energies, balancing the body inside and out. If you are older, incorporate more of the Panax or Siberian ginseng and if you are younger incorporate more of the astragalus.

   Recommended dose: 100–300 mg daily.

► Asian, Chinese, or Korean ginseng (*Panax ginseng*) and American Ginseng (*Panax quinquefolius*). From time immemorial, the Chinese have believed that ginseng is a cure for all diseases. The word ginseng is said to mean "the wonder of the world" and panax means "panacea." The properties of these ginsengs are similar to those of Siberian ginseng, but they are more potent. The mental and physical anti-fatigue effects of ginseng have been established in human clinical trials. Ginseng is a powerful adaptation that invigorates the whole system.

When buying ginseng root it is important to know the different types of ginseng, otherwise chances are that you will pay high prices for inferior qualities – unless you have a reputable source. Even in the health food store and herbal markets you need to be careful. Studies conducted on the quality of ginseng found that sixty percent of the "ginseng" products tested had little or no ginseng in them at all. Buy only from a company that you trust.

You should also realize that different varieties of ginseng will have different effects on your body. American ginseng contains the same active ingredients as *Panax ginseng* but in different proportions. American ginseng tends to depress the central nervous system, increase cholesterol synthesis in the liver and lower blood pressure. *Panax ginseng* slightly stimulates the central nervous system, increases blood pressure, is anabolic (i.e., stimulates protein and lipid synthesis), and may be responsible for increased body weight and enhanced resynthesis of glycogen and high energy compounds. Both tend to support the adrenal glands.

Ginseng contains many active ingredients including ginsenosides, panaquilon, saponins, panaxin, ginsenin and panoxic acid, to name a few. Panaquilon is a general endocrine tonic and performs a regulatory action on this system. It also affects the adrenal hormones which regulate many of our metabolic and adaptive functions. The saponins affect sugar metabolism, ginsenin acts somewhat like insulin, and panoxic acid regulates metabolism and the cardiovascular system, and prevents cholesterol build-up. Ginseng has also been shown to affect the thyroid gland.

Recommended dose: 2–4 g daily, increasing to 4–6 g daily one week before a race and for one or two days after. I recommend taking ginseng for three weeks then stopping for two weeks before resuming use.

► Siberian Ginseng *(Eleutherococcus senticosis)*. This is one of the most valuable adaptogens in the herbal kingdom. Japanese studies dating back to the 1980s have shown that aerobic capacity, heart rate, maximum work capacity and endurance improved in people taking Siberian ginseng. An increase in glycogen synthesis and a decrease in carbohydrate use was also noted.

It has been suggested that Siberian ginseng supports blood sugar levels which would give the brain more fuel and therefore enable a more efficient performance. Siberian ginseng supports the adrenocortical system that regulates the chemistry of stress. This system must be intact to resist the onset of stress-related fatigue.

Siberian ginseng's benefits are widely known. Regular ginseng use improves general health, memory and longevity. Olympic athletes, particularly from the former Soviet countries, routinely include adaptogenic herbs in their nutrition programs to give them a competitive edge.

Siberian ginseng contains eleutherocides (not ginsenosides), and it is a pure adaptogenic herb that restores homeostasis to the body (e.g., if blood pressure is high it will lower it, if blood pressure is low it will raise it). Siberian ginseng is The Great Normalizer.

Recommended dose: 2–4 ml of the fluid extract three times daily, or 200 mg of root powder three times daily.

I recommend that the Siberian ginseng be taken for two months followed by a two week break before starting another two month course. The dose can be increased two weeks before a race or any other demanding event.

- Brazilian Ginseng, Suma (*Pfaffia paniculata*). The urban Brazilians named this herb *para todo* meaning "for everything." This adaptogen is very powerful in combating the negative physiological effects of stress. Brazilian ginseng contains significant amounts of germanium which is involved in cell oxygenation. It has stimulating effects on the body and also contains beta-carotene, vitamins B_I, B_2 and E, potassium, and a full spectrum of essential amino acids.

Recommended dose: 1–4 g daily.

- Condonopsitis *(Condonopsitis radix)*. Also known as cordyceps sinensis, condonopsitis can be taken daily as a nutrient supplement. The well-known natural adaptogen is made from the *dong chong xia cao* worm – a fungus, not a worm – that grows on the wormlike larvae of certain moths. Condonopsitis is used in much the same manner as ginseng, but is not nearly as expensive. Chinese researchers claim that it can increase physical and mental endurance and is therefore excellent for athletes.

Recommended dose: The general recommendation is to take two 200 mg capsules daily.

- Licorice Root. There are two types of licorice root: western (*Glycyrrhiza glabra*) and Chinese (*Glycyrrhiza uralensis*). Western licorice root sometimes causes nervousness or gastrointestinal problems unlike the Chinese licorice which is calming, energizing and without side-effects. Studies on the western licorice root often involve the deglycyrrhizinated licorice (DGL) which seems to be free from side-effects. Include Chinese licorice or the deglycyrrhizinated western licorice as part of your health program.

Chinese licorice is the most widely used of all the Chinese herbs. It detoxifies your system, regulates your blood sugar levels, and the Chinese claim that it will build muscle. Athletes should note that licorice has the ability to increase glucocorticoids (adrenal hormones). This is particularly important when your blood sugar level drops following vigorous physical exertion.

Licorice root has a profound effect on the adrenal glands and helps maintain proper electrolyte balance in organ tissues. Although most products use glycyrrhizin licorice, a number of products use DGL. The latter form is used in the treatment of peptic ulcers. The active components of DGL are flavonoids – a group of compounds that have antioxidant properties and anti-inflammatory effects.

Licorice root can be taken in many forms. You can buy the Chinese roots and just chew them or make a tea and drink two or three cups throughout the day. Athletes who train two or more hours daily should prepare a tea made with Chinese licorice root and condonopsitis and use it in their water bottles for sustained energy.

Recommended dose: 350–500 mg of powdered root three times daily, or 2–4 ml of fluid extract three times daily.

► Sarsaparilla *(Smilax officinalis)*. In the US, *Smilax* has been used as a sexual rejuvenator and energy booster. Although sarsaparilla itself does not contain testosterone, the saponin in the plant can be transformed in the lab to testosterone. It has been shown to improve stamina, increase the oxidative-reduction process of the tissues (i.e., it will allow you to exercise longer before lactic acid build-up), enhance recovery after exercise and help balance the cardiovascular system.

Recommended dose: 2–4 ml of the fluid extract three times daily, or 250 mg of powdered sarsaparilla three times daily.

▸ Schizandra *(Schizandra chinensis)*. This is a very special herb and has been highly regarded by Chinese physicians for centuries. Its fame in China is due to its reputation as a beautifier, a sexual tonic, and a preserver of youth. Schizandra was found to reduce fatigue, enhance physical and mental performance, increase endurance, sharpen senses, improve general strength even during states of exhaustion, and relieves sexual fatigue and increase staying power in men.

Recommended dose: When preparing this herb, soak a handful in water for four to six hours. Throw out the water and rinse the herb, then add three cups of water, some licorice root and simmer gently for fifteen minutes. Drink daily for at least four months to build energy and superb stamina. The recommended dose for raw schizandra is 1–2 g daily. Schizandra is usually found in combination with other herbs in capsule or tincture form.

I have mentioned the most widely studied adaptogenic herbs and would strongly recommend that you incorporate two or three of these into your daily health program. If you are not sure which herbs or nutritional supplements to take, seek the advice of a naturopathic physician or other health care practitioner trained in complementary medicine.

TONIC HERBS

Tonic herbs are also of extreme importance in the physiological support of the body for both the beginner and elite athlete. Tonic herbs improve the assimilation of nutrients which in turn increases the energy and strength of the body. Each tonic herb has an affinity with a specific organ.

Of the tonic herbs, a number of plants supply steroidal saponins – anabolic steroid *precursors* (not anabolic steroids themselves) which the body can use to manufacture growth hormones. Steroidal saponins are the building blocks used by the body to produce its own steroids and as a result they are neither harmful to the liver nor are they banned in sports medicine. Banned substances are discussed later in this chapter.

▸ Licorice – western *(Glycyrrhiza glabra)* and Chinese *(Glycyrrhiza uralensis)*. See Adaptogenic Herbs earlier in this chapter.

▸ Sarsaparilla *(Smilax officinalis)*. See Adaptogenic Herbs earlier in this chapter.

▸ Wild Yam *(Dioscorea villosa)*. Most species of yam contain steroid precursors (not steroids), primarily diosgenin, which is needed for the synthesis of progesterone.

Recommended dose: 15–25 drops of wild yam tincture three times daily.

▸ Ginkgo *(Ginkgo biloba)*. Ginkgo is commonly used to treat poor circulation to the extremities, ringing in the ears, and memory loss associated with aging and the early stages of Alzheimer's disease. Of special interest to the athlete is its effect on the cardiovascular system. Ginkgo increases blood flow and oxygen circulation throughout the entire body and improves mental alertness. Ginkgo is also an antioxidant that rids the body of free radicals which are rapidly produced during training when oxidation rates are high. (See Antioxidants in Chapter 11).

Recommended dose of 24% ginkgolides (a standardized product): 40 mg three times daily or 20 drops of tincture three times daily.

CHINESE HERBAL MEDICINES

The scope of Chinese medicine is far too vast to cover in any detail in this book. I do, however, want to mention the use of specific herbs that are of particular interest to the athlete.

The philosophy of Chinese medicine is based on the flow of the *chi* (energy) through the body along channels called "meridians." Each meridian is directly connected to a specific organ.

When the flow of *chi* is interrupted in a specific meridian, the corresponding organ does not receive its full measure of energy and therefore will not function at its optimum level. *Chi* is further characterized as having yin and yang qualities.

For example, the Chinese "earth" element, which builds strong muscle, is governed by the spleen (yin) and stomach (yang) meridians in Chinese medicine. If the earth element is weak, your body becomes tired, sluggish, it will retain water, and digestive and blood disorders can occur. Your mind becomes foggy and depressed as well. Herbs such as Chinese licorice root, condonopsitis, and astragalus support the spleen and stomach meridians.

The liver (yin) and gall-bladder (yang) meridians govern the tendons and ligaments and control neuro-muscular activity. The liver and gall-bladder represent the "wood" element. If this element is out of balance your will becomes weak, you become irritable, angry, lethargic and even depressed. The liver is responsible for muscular tone and motor activity. Muscle tension is a result of an imbalance in the nervous system and therefore represents a liver imbalance in Chinese medicine.

Herbs which support the liver and gall-bladder are Lycii Fructus (*Lycium chinensis*), an excellent tonic that is easily obtained; Ho Shou Wu *(Polygonum multiflorum)* an excellent energy tonic that builds strength in the liver, kidneys, muscles and bones; and schizandra, as mentioned earlier, is also an excellent liver tonic and general adaptogen.

The kidney (yin) and bladder (yang) meridian includes the adrenals and is said to store the "vital essence" of life. Most tonic and adaptogenic herbs mentioned

ELEMENTS	YIN ORGAN	YANG ORGAN
Fire	Heart	Small Intestine
Earth	Spleen	Stomach
Metal	Lungs	Large Intestine
Water	Kidney	Bladder
Wood	Liver	Gall-bladder

In Chinese medicine these pairs are called "husband and wife" and they support each other when one of the organ systems is weak or congested.

stimulate this meridian. Low kidney *chi* can result in memory problems, backache, fatigue, poor concentration, joint inflammations, injury proneness, and decreased resistance to disease.

Cordyceps sinensis is a very important herb for the athlete. It is a restorative tonic and is the equivalent of ginseng for invigorating and toning the body. It is an excellent tonic for the lungs and kidneys. The price of cordyceps has increased significantly in the last few years, perhaps because of its increased popularity among Japanese and Chinese athletes. I recommend you make it into a tea (use about ten slices to two quarts/liters of water and simmer for one half hour) or a soup (use approximately ten slices for each pot of soup). The Chinese traditionally add cordyceps to chicken soup. I have found cordyceps to be equally as effective in vegetable soup.

Please note, if you have difficulty finding any of the Chinese or western herbs mentioned in this book, you can contact The Integrative Health Centre in Calgary (403) 228-1907 for assistance and recommendations.

ILLEGAL AND SYNTHETIC ERGOGENICS

As long as we remain competitive and drive ourselves to new heights, it is natural to want to find ways to maximize our efforts. Many of us do this in the form of proper eating, quality rest and recovery, smart training programs and visualization. Yet as you approach your limits, the temptation to reach higher levels by using synthetic ergogenics can be overwhelming. You should be aware of the dangers of these substances and know that there is no substitute for optimum performance achieved naturally.

Given that we have limited time or sometimes feel we just cannot train anymore without risk of injury, the "ergogenic industry" offers us that little extra help from performance-enhancing drugs. Ergogenics is a broad term for substances that enhance performance. This is not something new; the ancient Greeks and Romans made use of such substances. They believed that by eating certain animal organs they would improve their performance. Many cultures still subscribe to such beliefs. Chinese pharmacies offer a wide arrangement of unusual animal products with esoteric healing properties. Among the products you might find are deer antler, seahorse, gecko and bear gall-bladder. A number of nutrition companies (mostly European) use such products in their medicines. I have experimented with several of these products in the past, but out of concern for animals and the quality of the product I discontinued their use and now only use natural ergogenics.

Many ergogenic aids are both safe and legal. Yet there are many illegal ergogenic aids and these usually involve pharmacological products. While they can provide certain short-term benefits, they can be extremely dangerous to one's health. If you subscribe to our philosophy of natural health, you will avoid all synthetic substances.

A survey by a member of the US Olympic Drug Control Program recently found that approximately ninety percent of male weight lifters, power lifters and bodybuilders from various health clubs had used steroids, while another study found that thirty-eight percent of high school football players and twenty percent of other high school athletes used banned ergogenic substances.

"Doping," or the use of illegal substances by athletes in attempts to enhance their performance has a long history, but it wasn't until the 1960 Olympic Games in Rome, after the death of a cyclist who had illegal drugs in his system, that the International Olympic Committee (IOC) adopted strong measures to govern anti-doping legislation. Since then, most other major sporting organizations have followed suit but their impact has been comparably marginal. Coaches and athletes continue to find new drugs and new ways of beating the drug testing system thereby gaining an edge over other athletes. In fact, virtually no major sporting event has avoided a doping scandal.

USER BEWARE

Silken Laumann, one of Canada's greatest rowers, cost her rowing team the gold medal at the 1995 Pan-American Games in Argentina after she tested positive for the banned stimulant pseudophedrine. The banned substance was in a cold remedy recommended by the team doctor even after Laumann had asked several times whether or not it was on the IOC list of banned substances.

If you wish to compete, be very careful about taking any kind of over-the-counter or prescription drug. If the substance is in any way medicative then do *not* use it unless it is prescribed by your physician. This should be your number one rule – especially if you're using it for the first time at a race. If you do require medication, check first with local medical experts or sports council officials as to whether the drug is, or contains, a banned substance. In addition to the serious side-effects of anabolic steroids, most banned substances detract from, rather than enhance, performance.

Triathlon has had its share of athletes using illegal ergogenics. Since most triathletes are not interested in building bulk, the issue of taking too much protein or any other bodybuilding stimulant is seldom discussed in the triathlon literature. Whether you want a more defined body, a weight change or an improvement in strength, power and endurance, you might be tempted to experiment with growth hormone stimulants. Pantothenic acid, calcium pantothenate, and amino acids such as arginine and ornithine, are available over the counter. Many growth stimulants, however, are not. The latter generally come in the form of anabolic steroids – the "win at all costs" drugs. While you need to be very careful about the type and dose of "legal" human growth stimulants you take, the illegal stimulants can be deadly.

WHAT ARE ANABOLIC STEROIDS?

Anabolic steroids are synthetic variations of testosterone. They provide dramatic shortcuts to improved speed, strength and muscle mass. As we will see however, the side-effects are *deadly*.

Aside from cheating yourself and fellow competitors, the most important reason for staying away from anabolic steroids (AS) is the potential lifelong harm you can inflict on yourself for the sake of a few moments of fame. Former football great, Lyal Alzato admitted to taking AS and paid the price for his enhanced performance with his life. After being diagnosed with brain cancer brought on by overuse of AS, he dedicated what little was left of his life to warning others of the dangers of these stimulants.

Without going into detail, some of the more commonly-documented health risks found to be associated with anabolic steroids include:

▸ *Reproductive system risks.* Anabolic steroids affect the male reproductive system by shutting down natural testosterone production. Prolonged use may lead to such problems as sterility and enlarged breasts. For women, prolonged use may result in androgen-related body changes such as the loss of breasts, deeper voices, facial hair, enlarged clitoris, acne, menstrual irregularities and an array of other side-effects which can become permanent.

▸ *Cardiovascular damage.* You may have heard that former NHL star John Kordic died from heart failure as a result of using anabolic steroids. Lesser side-effects include elevated blood pressure and irregular heart beat. The metabolism of fats and sugars can be affected by anabolic steroids in such a way that it leads to fatty deposits in the heart which can result in heart attacks.

▸ *Psychological problems.* Numerous studies note that anabolic steroid users experience severe mood swings, paranoia and elevated tendencies toward aggressive behavior. Prolonged use can lead to aggression, depression, permanent personality changes and even attempts at suicide.

▸ *Other common side-effects.* These include kidney failure, liver problems, weakening of connective tissue (increases the risk of injury), water retention and loss of appetite.

MORE ON OVER- AND UNDER-THE-COUNTER "DRUGS"

Drug testing is becoming the norm rather than the exception in most established sports. Most athletes are really unaware as to what constitutes an acceptable versus an unacceptable drug. After all, there are no rules saying you cannot smoke while racing, or for that matter put beer, wine or spirits in your water bottle and yet these substances can have temporary physiological effects such as numbing pain or providing a false sense of well-being. Furthermore, knowing which drugs are considered acceptable is not necessarily a matter of common sense.

The list of banned substances is extensive and many of these are readily obtainable in grocery and drug stores. Everything from sleeping pills to coffee and most cold remedies contain banned substances. You must also be aware that many banned substances have tolerance limits. That is, you must have a certain amount of the banned substance in your body in order to test positive. Therefore, while one cup of coffee may be fine, three cups could put you over the acceptable limit for caffeine. For someone who seldom drinks coffee, however, one cup may give them that extra edge that a regular coffee drinker would not notice.

While the list of banned substances is extensive, there are eight which are common in over-the-counter products.

▸ *Caffeine.* Commonly found in headache tablets, muscle relaxants, sleeping pills, coffee and most soft drinks.

▸ *Ephedrine.* An ingredient in many cold remedies. You should check all nasal decongestants because the legal standards for the allowable amounts may vary from country to country.

- *Desoxyephedrine.* Often found in nasal sprays.

- *Ma Huang.* A herbal ephedrine found in a variety of American performance supplements. Many herbal teas also contain traces of Ma Huang. Most of these teas are not available in Canada but if the tea promises any form of energy enhancement it is wise to read the list of ingredients carefully.

- *Phenyleprine/phenylpropanolamine/propylhexdrine/pseudophedrine.* These products are found in a variety of cold, nasal, allergy and hay fever remedies.

BLOOD DOPING

Beyond banned substances there is also blood doping. In essence, blood doping involves using a blood transfusion to improve your tolerance of low oxygen levels. Blood that is rich in red blood cells is injected into the athlete shortly before an event. The enriched red blood cell count delays the onset of fatigue. Although recognized for some time, blood doping only became a major issue at the 1976 Montreal Summer Olympics and was finally banned in 1985. Unfortunately, however, no reliable test is available to detect its use.

The bottom line is: the more familiar you can be with banned substances, the more you should be able to train and race clean. If you have any questions about an ergogenic product, you can contact:

The Canadian Sports Medicine and Science Council of Canada
1600 James Naismith Drive
Suite 502
Gloucester, ON K1B 5N4
(613) 748–5671

In the United States contact:

The American College of Sports Medicine
P.O. Box 1440
Indianapolis, IN 46206
(317) 637–9200

In Canada, you can also check the *Controlled Drugs and Illegal Substances Act* of 1996 in the *Criminal Code*. American athletes should consult the *Narcotic Control Act* and the *Controlled Substance Act* as well as the American *Criminal Code*. If you have any doubt about a substance – do not use it!

There is little pride in winning or excelling when you know you have cheated. While no one else may ever know, it is your conscience that will have to face the truth.

Chapter 15

Peaking: Getting Prepared for Competition

It is uncanny how many athletes I meet who, in doing their "homework," neglect one essential element of the package – mastering the before and after aspects of competing. That is, knowing not only how to train but how to taper for an event and what to do after the race. In this chapter we will explain what you need to know about race preparation, racing strategies, transitions and post-race recovery, as well as the importance of stretching.

· Even though you want to "kick butt," racing should always be fun and promote good health.

· Since training is not the same as racing, you should not approach the race as just another workout.

· The satisfaction of completing a race in inclement weather can be exhilarating.

· Racing is about winning within yourself.

TAPERING

Tapering your training is a very important part of your pre-race strategy. You have worked hard to prepare for the event and now you need to bring it all together. Since training is not the same as racing you must not approach the race as "just another workout." For many athletes this is very difficult because they are so disciplined in their training that to skip a beat is considered a fault!

Some of the questions I am regularly asked are: To what degree do I need to taper? How often do I need to taper? Won't

I lose my conditioning and competitive edge? Many coaches and programs recommend doing nothing but rest for several days before the event, and then doing a light workout the day before the race. This helps to calm your nerves and to get you mentally prepared. If you have been training all year, you will not lose your conditioning by taking it easy during the tapering phase, on the contrary, you will allow your body to build up some energy reserves.

One week before a big race, I start cutting my training volume by twenty-five percent *each day* while keeping the workouts intense. Three days before a big race I do nothing but rest; in the last two days I train very lightly. But I'm not really *training* during this time; rather I exercise to cut the tension and keep the blood flowing. On the other hand, I know some top triathletes who will do the whole riding course and maybe half the running course the day before just to get psyched.

Remember, above all, even though you want to "kick butt," racing should always be fun and ultimately promote good overall health.

Since your body has become used to your training routine, any major changes you make the week before a big race are not likely to feel comfortable. Therefore, your tapering phase should not be too different from your regular training program. There are, however, some important considerations:

▸ The week before the race, you should cut down on your meat consumption since your body does not need the protein at this time and meat takes too much energy to digest.

▸ Your weekly training volume should drop markedly – how much depends on the length of the race and your ability to rest. Being aware that any extra training will not enhance your performance (use the TRIMPS formula to objectively reduce your volume of training). If the race is an Ironman, then a three to four week tapering schedule can be very effective. For

Olympic-distance events a three to four day taper often suffices. Again, such tapers should be dictated by frequency of racing, intensity of training and importance of the race for you. For the World Masters Games in 1994, I began a modified tapering program three weeks before the short course event and as a result I produced my best ever swim and run times.

▶ Practice positive visualization. Mentally rehearse the race and your performance. See yourself doing well and thriving on the challenge rather than your placing. Recall other successful races or challenges. This not only reminds you that you are capable of doing well but it also floods your body with endorphins and reduces physical stress. An old sports adage says the difference between winning and losing is often ninety-nine percent mental.

The degree to which your performance is diminished is directly affected by your level of conditioning. Decline in performance during exercise layoff varies from sport to sport but as a general rule, the decline is most dramatic during the first two weeks. In *Galloway's Book on Running*, Jeff Galloway measures the decline in performance during exercise drop-off and offers the following chart to gauge the amount of conditioning you will lose during periods of inactivity.

Table 15.1 EFFECTS OF EXERCISE LAYOFF

Rest time without any exercise (days)	Estimated percent of conditioning lost
1–5	0–1
7	10
14	35
21	60
28	85
more than 35 days	100

RACE STRATEGIES

Once you have picked the races in which you would like to compete, you should then plan backwards. Yes, if you are racing, plan your training schedule around your race season. If you have been leading an active lifestyle allow yourself six to eight weeks to sufficiently prepare for Olympic-distance triathlons or duathlons that take less than two hours.

Six to eight weeks before the first race of your race season, establish your benchmark fitness level. Either pick some local swim, bike and running events, or go out and time yourself over a fixed distance which is the same distance as the upcoming race. Now, if you plan on doing both short- and long-distance races, stick to the short and middle distances when testing yourself.

Assuming you have been staying active all year, you will have an idea as to your desired race pace. For example, you might want to run 6-minute miles (1,600 meters) in a short course. Run at that pace, note how you feel and monitor your heart rate. Keep this information for future reference. Similarly, if you plan on swimming a 22-minute 1,500 meter race, then try to hold that pace when you are timing yourself. If you are able to complete the test events in the desired time without spending the entire time in your anaerobic zone, then your goals are realistic. See Table 15.2 for short-course average race paces. For example, if you can swim 100 meters in two minutes, you should be able to swim 1.5 km in 30 minutes. Or, if you can sustain a cycling pace of about thirty-eight km per hour, you ought to be able to cycle 40 km in 63 minutes. These figures will help you gauge your finish time in each of these events.

Table 15.2 SHORT-COURSE AVERAGE RACE PACE

SWIM		BIKE		RUN	
time (min) per 1.5 km	time (min) per 100 m	time (min) per 40 km	av. speed (km/hr)	time (min) per 10 km	av. speed (km/hr)
40	2:40	90	26.2	55:54	5.55
35	2:20	85	28.2	49:42	4.94
30	2:00	80	30.6	45:34	4.33
24	1:36	70	33.4	41:26	4.12
23	1:32	65	36.9	39:22	3.92
22	1:28	63	38.1	36:14	3.61
21	1:24	61	39.3	34:10	3.41
20	1:20	59	40.7	33:08	3.30
17	1:08	57	42.1	32:06	3.20
less than 17 – you're fast!		55	43.5	31:04	3.10

Keep your regular training program the same, but start to add some more intervals to your schedule. For short-course events these intervals can include swimming 50–200 m sprints; running 200–800 m sprints and cycling 400–1,000 m sprints. All intervals should be done at your desired racing heart rate. Proper warm-ups are essential.

About three weeks before the race season begins, you may want to include regular weekly massages and chiropractic visits to help keep you supple and to ensure your body is properly aligned. Massage should not be a substitute for regular stretching – it simply ensures that any problem areas can either be worked out or contained.

Given how close you are to the race, and given the volume of training you have already completed, do not add any workouts or attempt to increase your distances or improve your time. If you have been following your program, you have all the training you need. The key is knowing when you are ready and then concentrating on doing your best.

Starting two weeks before your race, take about ten to twenty minutes, three to four times weekly, to visualize the race. Your visualization should include being relaxed, racing smoothly and strongly throughout the event. *Visualize* the course (the hills, hairpin turns) making smooth transitions, and having a strong finish. If you can, check out the actual race course – it will help to prepare you for the competition. Roger Bannister, the first runner to break the legendary four-minute mile barrier, visualized the entire race scenario before his 1953 historic run in Vancouver's Empire Stadium. It sometimes takes a major shift in belief before we can achieve our goals.

A number of years ago, I participated in a half-Ironman distance race that included a bizarre set of corners and switchbacks in the last 2–3 kilometers of the run. While I had checked out the entire bike course and seen the unusual swim course, I did not bother with the running course, assuming it would be fairly straightforward as it had been described as a flat out-and-back course. At kilometer seventeen the leader took a wrong turn on the rather poorly marked course. As he was just out of earshot, I was unable to inform him of his mistake. When I turned onto the proper route I could see the former lead runner turn around and head back. I had my own problems though: not being familiar with the course, I had difficulty pacing myself over the final 2–3 kilometers and I had no idea how far I was from the finish. At the same time the fellow behind was intent on making up lost ground. I managed to prevail, but it was a tainted victory. The second place finisher and I had neglected to familiarize ourselves with the course. Don't let this happen to you!

What to do a week before the race is a matter of controversy. In the past, coaches recommended taking it easy and cutting back on the volume and intensity of your training. They also recommended you alter your diet to include more complex carbohydrates. Today, most experts have moved away from these recommendations. Gale Bernhardt, who coaches triathletes and duathletes, and contributes to *Triathlete* magazine, recommends maintaining the intensity of the training in the last week but cutting back on the volume. According to her formula, the last week should contain only fourteen percent of the volume you did three weeks earlier. She recommends cutting back to sixty percent of your normal training volume three weeks before, then cutting back to forty percent of your training volume two weeks before the race.

This formula is a general guideline, and, as usual, we recommend you tailor your own tapering program based on your feelings and performance. As has been noted earlier, no magic formula exists. Cutting back too much can cause you to get stale, and maintaining too high a carbohydrate diet may cause you to gain weight and feel lethargic. Wheat-based products (e.g., pasta and bread) tend to have an alkalizing effect and make you feel sluggish.

Monitoring your heart rate will remind you to stay aerobic and not to spend too much time in your anaerobic zone. A few

MENTAL FITNESS TEST

1. Do I see the relationship between my state of mind and my ability to perform?

2. Will competition make me perform better?

3. Have I visualized the race course as completely as possible?

4. Have I visualized myself running, swimming and cycling smoothly and effortlessly?

5. Do I view the challenge of competition as fun?

6. Am I prepared to do my best – even if the conditions are unfavorable?

7. Do I look for ways to refine and improve my performance?

8. Am I able to maintain my concentration and stick to my program during the stress and excitement of racing?

9. Has my training program helped me to prepare for the race?

10. Do I have the support of family and friends?

11. Has my commitment to a healthy lifestyle changed my life for the better?

12. Do my present abilities match my expectations?

13. Can I turn pre-race tension to good account?

TO PEAK OR NOT TO PEAK?

If you plan on doing several races throughout the season, you might want to pick two or three in which you would like to do your best. To perform at your full potential in every race is almost impossible. Even those racers who win everything and who race year-round are not peaking for every race. In fact, during those periods when they race a lot, many will simply train lightly between races – they use the times in-between races as active recovery periods. Just as world-class cyclist Miguel Induráin focuses his year around the Tour de France, or Mark Allen around the Nice Triathalon and the Ironman triathlons, other racers focus on a few key races in which they can do their best.

Many amateur duathletes and triathletes try to race almost every weekend, especially those in the northern climates where the race season can be short. In order to survive a short season you need to prioritize your races. Perhaps you want to do well at the provincial or state championships, the Nationals or the Worlds. The years I planned such a season, I would do mini-peaks and race only hard enough to make it to the Worlds where I would lay it all out.

anaerobic accelerations in any sport are fine, but they should not be sustained efforts.

On the final few days before a big race some athletes prefer to do nothing. Others like to do a light workout the day before the race and take the second last day off completely – the couch potato day. I used to copy what others did and would veg out for two days before each Ironman and drink fluids and carbo load as if I were preparing for a survival event. Then, as I began to tailor my own program, my routine changed dramatically.

While it is generally wise not to overdo it the last few days, you need to find the balance of rest and light activity that suits your needs. Only race experience, however, will determine what works best for you. Keep a detailed record of the final week of training leading up to your key races, monitor how you feel on race day *and* the quality of your performance. Remember: nothing is constant. As we age, our pre-race preparation is likely to change.

RACE RULES

1. Before leaving the first transition (swim-to-bike), your helmet must be on and fastened before mounting your bike.

2. Most races require you to walk your bike out of the transition area. You are not allowed to mount your bike in the transition zone – no matter how far away you are from the start line! This is done for safety reasons.

3. At most races, you have to return your bike to its proper place and remount it on the racks. Therefore, remember where you got it.

4. After finishing the ride, remove your helmet last. Unfastening it before you dismount will result in a disqualification.

5. Many races require racers to have their chest covered before they enter the running course. Also, most races require racers to wear a top. Perhaps it's all in the name of equality – men could get an unfair cooling advantage over women.

If you intend to race, get a copy of the latest rules. They are usually available from your local, provincial, or regional triathlon/duathlon office.

RACE REMINDER CHECKLIST

Making sure you have all your equipment could be called racing's hidden transition. This may sound trite, but many an experienced racer can tell you horror stories of equipment left behind. Have you ever gone to work or gone on a holiday and forgotten something important? When the tension begins to mount just before the race, it can be helpful, even for the most seasoned athlete to rely on a checklist. Items in square brackets are optional.

SWIM:
- ☐ swimsuit(s)
- ☐ goggles: clean, leakproof [colored lenses for sun, extra pairs]
- ☐ wetsuit for open water swims
- ☐ lubricant (Vaseline™ or silicone spray)
- ☐ towel
- ☐ swimcap
- ☐ [sunscreen]
- ☐ [basin to rinse feet]
- ☐ [ear plugs, nose plugs]
- ☐ [goggle defog]

CYCLE:
- ☐ bicycle – *fully inspected*
- ☐ water bottles
- ☐ ANSI-approved helmet
- ☐ [sunglasses, eye protection]
- ☐ [air pump and/or air cartridges]
- ☐ [heart-rate monitor]
- ☐ [socks]
- ☐ spare wheels, tires, tubes
- ☐ cycling shoes
- ☐ [Vaseline™]
- ☐ [tool kit]
- ☐ [wind- and waterproof shell jacket]
- ☐ [cycling gloves]

RUN:
- ☐ running shoes w/zip ties
- ☐ shirt/singlet for men
- ☐ [sun/rain hat]
- ☐ [heart-rate monitor]
- ☐ [socks]
- ☐ shorts
- ☐ [sunglasses]
- ☐ [lightweight gloves]

OTHER:
- ☐ [sports drinks for long races]
- ☐ shower gear for post-race shower and change of clothes
- ☐ post-race food/nutrition
- ☐ bag for essentials: keys, wallet, ID, access passes and water
- ☐ [watch]
- ☐ [energy bars for long rides/runs]
- ☐ sports bag for gear
- ☐ [heart-rate monitor]

JUST IN CASE:
- ☐ registration form
- ☐ support crew
- ☐ map/directions to race

TRIATHLON TRANSITION TIPS

The key to good transitions is to practice the routine. Try different approaches and time them. How can you best remove your wetsuit? Are you better off remaining standing or sitting while you change over? Good transitions can save valuable time which in short races may make a significant difference in the final placement. The following section summarizes in point form what you need to do to execute successful changeovers in a triathlon. Each transition is then discussed in more detail below.

Table 15.3 TRIATHLON TRANSITION TIPS

The Swim

- Remember where your cycling gear is. Use some kind of orientation point.
- Do you have an appropriate lubricant to help remove your wetsuit?
- Goggles. Are the straps adjusted, the lenses clear and the fit proper?
- Seed yourself according to your speed. If you are a moderately
  fast swimmer, do not go to the front or stay in the back.

Swim-to-Bike Transition

- Breathe deeply and relax as you change into your riding gear. Follow a practised sequence. Perhaps put your shoes on first then your sunglasses, etc.
- Have all your cycling equipment organized and ready. For example, your velcro straps should be open and your helmet strap unlocked.
- Your bike should be set up in a relatively easy gear.
- Most races now require you to walk your bike out of the transition to the start line.
- Fasten your helmet before you mount your bike.
- Once you mount your bike, spend the first few minutes in an easier gear until you feel your legs have properly adjusted.

Bike-to-Run Transition

- Just before finishing the ride (for the last 500 m), stand and stretch your hamstrings and calves. A few seconds lost on the bike will quickly be gained on the run.
- Remember where your orientation point is when you return your bike to start the run.
- Do not remove your helmet before you are off your bike.
- Have your running attire laid out and ready.
- Again, start the run with short and more conservative strides until your legs get used to the running motion.

SWIM-TO-BIKE TRANSITION

Even though the changeover from swimming to biking is the least stressful of the transitions, it can be disorienting. Since you are switching from upper body to lower body muscle groups the muscles may not feel taxed, but going from a horizontal to a vertical position as quickly as you can might produce a slight sense of confusion. Watch how swimmers exit the water, remove their wetsuits and move onto their bikes. It is not difficult to spot the beginners. Practice removing your wetsuit a number of times. If you are inexperienced, it can become a frustrating task in the rush of the race.

Just before you exit the water (last 15–20 meters or so), change your stroke to tell your body that it will soon be expected to do something different. A few breast strokes or back crawl strokes will remove some of the pooled blood and help your mind to switch gears. The few seconds you might lose can often be made up on the bike or run sections with little difficulty. Mentally rehearse what you need to do when getting out of the water. Where is your bike gear? Where is your bike? Do you need to pass off a swim tag? Do you need to wash off any sand? (It is no fun cycling with sand in your shoes – and those blisters will get even bigger on the run.) Do you need to change clothes? Where is your change bag?

These reminders might sound silly, but when your bike is among a sea of 2,000 other bikes, being aware and prepared can make a big difference. I always look for key landmarks to orient myself. If there are a lot of participants, I will often physically rehearse the swim-to-bike transition before having to leave the transition zone. I have seen too many other athletes get lost at this stage. Not only did they lose time, but being unable to locate their equipment produced unnecessary stress.

As you get out of the water, keep moving but do not panic.

Race at your pace – dictate your own speed and go through your transition as quickly but as calmly as you can. If possible, sit down when putting on your cycling shoes unless they are already on your pedals. If they are, be sure you are used to entering your shoes this way. I lost valuable time at a big race while trying this time-saving method for the first time without ever having practiced it. I ran into a fence and fell off my bike trying to get my feet into the shoes. In the off-season you can practice and see which technique works best for you.

Before you actually race, try a number of different transition combinations. Are you more efficient with all your gear by your bike? Is it more efficient to place your helmet on top of your bars? Should you put it on last? Is it best to leave your shoes in the pedals? Only experimentation will tell. Whatever you do, practice so that it becomes second nature.

When starting out on the bike, it is usually best to start in a slightly easier gear (small ring in front and the third ring on the rear cog: 42-15/16) until your legs – especially your quadriceps and hamstrings – have adjusted to the change. They should adapt fairly quickly and then you can go for it.

BIKE-TO-RUN TRANSITION

Over the final 300–500 meters get out of the saddle and stretch your legs, calves and lower back. This is very helpful when you are competing in long distance races. Shake your legs and pedal backwards for twenty or so revolutions to relieve some of the blood pooling in your legs. Slowing down also lets your heart rate recover a little. The stretching will allow you to begin the run looking less like a duck than you might actually feel. A few seconds of slowing down will give you time to anticipate your transition with a calm, cool attitude. Make sure you remember where your orientation point is – and do not remove your helmet until you are off your bike.

Other important considerations are: Do you need to return your bike during the transition or will someone do it for you? (Some racing rules prohibit support staff from returning your bike.) Where is your change of clothes? (These should be laid out and ready.) Where is the running start? Do you need to drink some water?

After placing your bike, sit down and put your shoes on properly. As you leave the transition area you can put on your singlet and turn your race number around. Many racers like to put their race numbers on an elastic band so that they can show it on their back while cycling, and wear it on their front while running. Practice the bike-to-run transition a few times so that you can do it without running into other bikes.

Your running shoes should have elastic-type laces with pull toggles for easy entry and fastening. However, a few shoe models now have velcro-fastening systems. Some athletes have even had zippers installed in place of a lacing system. These devices all allow for quicker transitions since there are no laces to tie. A little Vaseline™ in the heels of your shoes can help your foot slip in more easily. Socks are your choice. They take time but may provide a little extra comfort – especially if you are running some dirt trails or doing a half- or full-Ironman distance race. You can roll your socks so that they are easier to put on. You might also consider applying a little baby powder beforehand to allay any rubbing from socks that are not on properly. Find out what works best for you and stick to it.

Start out the run segment with a short shuffling stride, and then as your legs feel comfortable and your heart rate is normal for you, put the hammer down. Go for it!

ENERGY LOADING

Regardless of the distance you are racing, your body can benefit from some complex carbohydrate loading. Even though you may be eating well throughout your training program, races are events that require special attention to details. Therefore, stop carbo-loading about eighteen hours before the race to allow sufficient time for your system to digest and store the energy as glycogen.

Carbohydrate loading can, however, cause you to gain weight. This is normal because water will be stored in the muscles along with the extra carbohydrates you have consumed. Some athletes will even increase their daily intake of complex carbohydrates to seventy percent of their total calories during this phase. You should avoid raw or difficult to digest foods (e.g., popcorn, fruit, raw veggies) while carbo-loading since you are usually in some state of stress during this period and your stomach won't be working as efficiently as usual. (If you have diabetes or hypertriglyceridemia and are considering carbo-loading, consult your physician).

Unless you are racing late in the day, the pre-race meal is not really necessary other than to keep your routine somewhat intact. It should be consumed at least three hours before the race.

You may find yourself needing to go to the bathroom several times before the race starts – the nerves do wonders for cleansing the system. (An interesting note from Chinese medicine: the kidneys are the organs that process and store fear.) Coffee, although a stimulant, can have a negative effect, especially if you have butterflies in your stomach, and it is a diuretic. Some people claim coffee helps them to clear their bowels before the race. Given the line-ups at the porto-johns on race day, I do not think many people have a problem in this area. Therefore, you are better off warming up for twenty to thirty minutes by going short distances at race pace. This will focus your mind and warm up your body better than a few extra cups of coffee. Go for the real thing!

FLUID LOADING

Our bodies are made up of approximately seventy percent water. Water transports nutrients, regulates body temperature and facilitates a number of other vital bodily functions. Therefore, adequate water intake is essential not only during training but during pre-race preparation as well. For two days before the race, be sure to take in lots of fluids – fifteen or more glasses of water or an electrolyte drink a day is good. If it is hot and humid, force yourself to drink even more. Your body will thank you for it. Several years ago at the World Triathlon Championships in Florida I neglected this basic rule and paid dearly for it over a short course. You want your body to be well hydrated. You will know your body is well hydrated when you urinate quite regularly and your urine is clear.

After an hour of intense exercise you will lose nearly 40 ounces (1.2 liters or 5 cups) of fluid! Matching fluid loss with fluid intake during intense competition is physiologically impossible because less than 24 ounces (0.70 liter or 3 cups) of fluids empties from the stomach during the stress of exercise. Therefore, *"superhydration"* is key to races lasting 60 minutes or more. (Many endurance races lasting twelve or more hours require you to stop for periodic weight checks. If your body weight drops below a predetermined percentage, you are required to withdraw. Dehydration can be very injurious.) Remember:

▶ *Do not rely on your thirst response.* If you do, it will be too late to adequately rehydrate yourself.

▶ Take any ergogenic aids (caffeine, calcium lactate, ginseng, etc.) at least two hours before competition. This will allow time for them to enter your blood and do their work. Please note that caffeine is only legal to a level of 12 micrograms per milliliter in the urine and its ergogenic effects are unpredictable.

▸ If the race requires flying or long-distance travel, go to the race site a few days early. In addition to adjusting to the environment it will allow you to properly hydrate. (Air travel tends to dehydrate your body.) I strongly recommend carrying your own water and food supply on board.

▸ Exercise at the coolest times of the day leading up to the race to prevent dehydration.

Research suggests that water loss up to three percent of your total body weight is fairly safe; five percent or less is borderline, while a loss of over seven percent can severely affect the functioning of the heart and circulatory system and if not corrected, could result in death. Dehydration also creates an electrolyte imbalance. Salt tablets or extra potassium should not be used to treat water loss (see Chapters 9 and 16). If you use a commercial energy drink then it should not contain more than 2.5 percent sugar per volume. The best ones will contain glucose polymers, fructose and maltodextrins as they are absorbed quickly and help maintain normal blood sugar levels. Studies have shown that as long as the concentration is between five to seven percent these drinks empty from the stomach only marginally slower than pure water.

During prolonged exercise, perspiration will not evaporate quickly enough to keep the body cool. Excessive fluid loss will raise your body's temperature and as a result your body will begin to shut down – quite a remarkable survival mechanism but your performance will drop dramatically and you may risk internal injuries. Unless you are well trained and live in hot regions, body functions start to be compromised at temperatures above 75°F (24°C) and relative humidity above fifty percent.

THE NIGHT BEFORE THE RACE

Virtually every training book will tell you that the most important night for getting sleep is two nights before the race. The anticipation and excitement of an important race usually give even the most seasoned racer a less than perfect last night's sleep. I usually do lots of easy stretching and watch television or read in a reclined position with my legs elevated. I will also do a last-minute check of all my equipment and gear. I get to bed before 10 PM and visualize the course and my race. I then block everything out of my mind and hunker down for a few hours of sleep. By 4 AM however, I'm usually awake and raring to go, and looking forward to having a fun and good race.

LAST MINUTE EQUIPMENT CHECK

You have taken good care of your body and it is ready to perform – but what about your equipment? You have been training and racing in and on it perhaps all year. Or maybe, you only bring out those special wheels, goggles and runners for the big races. Well, you want to make sure they do not let you down. Unless you are well versed in maintaining your racing equipment, have it professionally checked – especially your bike. It is a good idea to have everything checked during the final week leading up to the race.

Ideally, try to check your gear at least two days before the race. Are your goggles leak proof? Do you have a back-up pair? Is your wetsuit comfortable? If you haven't worn it recently, does it still fit you? Are your running shoes in order? Do you have all the necessary equipment for the race and transition area. Has your bike been checked: tires, brakes, seat post, gears and all locking devices (I once had my seat post come loose in a race because I had not bothered to check it – even though I had done a fair bit of rough road riding just a few days prior. I had to finish the last ten km out of the saddle). Do not rely on the mandatory bike check to catch these things. They usually just do the basics like checking to see if your brakes work, the tires are glued on properly and your headset is snug.

Do *not* plan to use any equipment that you are not used to. If you are fortunate enough to have more than one bike, or several pairs of running shoes, make sure you have tried them out and are comfortable with them. Do not, for example, decide to put a new set of aerobars or an advanced seat post on your bike, or switch to super lightweight runners, or buy a new wetsuit just before the race without using them a few times under simulated race conditions. If you are going to change anything, do it early in your training season to give your body time to adjust.

Chapter 16

Race Day

As with all other aspects of training and health, your race day should be comprised of rituals that are tailored for *you*. I like to get up early and stretch a little, check the weather, meditate briefly or do some t'ai chi. I usually go for a short jog (and dress more warmly than the weather calls for) to check all my systems. From this routine, I can get a good idea how the day will unfold. Then I have a shower and eat a light meal of toast, a healthy cereal with water, and perhaps drink a coffee along with more water. My pre-race routine is usually completed about one-and-a-half to two hours before the start of the race.

· Racing is about winning within yourself and knowing you did your best.

· Racing will reveal the relationship between your state of mind and your ability to perform.

Since my energy level is quite high, I avoid arriving too early at the start line. Knowledge of the number of participants and the organizational level of the race allow me to gauge the time of my arrival. Since I prefer to stay focused, I am not big on small talk and renewing friendships before the race – that is what the postrace period is about for me. Others, however, find it very relaxing to mingle. It is perhaps one of the differences between introverts like me and extroverts.

Check your bike one last time before the race. Many races require you to leave your bike at the site the night before. Check your tire pressure, put your bike into an easy gear, and organize your equipment to ensure smooth transitions from swim to bike to run. Set up your transition area. Keep an extra water bottle on hand during the pre-race period to stay hydrated. Get to the washroom line-up early – it can get long just before the gun goes off.

BEFORE THE RACE – WARM-UP

At my first race I couldn't believe that people were jogging or swimming before the gruelling event. When I saw one top German athlete riding a stationary trainer just before the start of the first Ironman Europe in 1988, I thought he was either showing off, trying to intimidate his opponents, or had simply had one too many of those renowned German beers the night before. Well, today virtually everyone does a pre-race warm-up. Most warm-ups are done fifteen to thirty minutes before the start of the race. This might involve a short one to two mile jog with a few wind sprints thrown in; a five to ten minute spin on a stationary trainer and the ritual plunge into the waters. One year, however, while participating in a race in Cold Lake, Alberta (the lake lived up to its name) not one athlete took the ritual pre-race swim warm-up. We all waded in and immediately questioned our sanity. The purpose of a good warm-up is to relieve a little tension, to elevate your heart rate slightly and to break a light sweat. When the gun goes off you want to be ready to go hard.

HYDRATION

About thirty minutes before the race drink eight to sixteen ounces of water (even though you may not be thirsty). This will delay dehydration. Drinking water should not be cold as your stomach does not absorb it as well as tepid water. This point is somewhat controversial. I suspect the reason some recommend drinking cold water is that it may go down easier – like a cool drink on a hot day. On the other hand, some people experience discomfort and headaches if they consume water that is too cold when the body is heated from racing. By the time race day rolls around, you should have already determined what works best for you.

During the race, drink about eight ounces of fluid every fifteen to twenty minutes. On the bike, you should consume about two bottles of water every hour – more if it is very humid. Do not rely on your thirst response. *If you start feeling thirsty, it is too late!* You will start to slow down and may have cramps. If you want or need to consume energy food, do so on the bike when your system is more able to digest and process such food than while running. Drink at least a little water (and more if you feel like it) at every aid station. Research on marathoners showed that runners had the most success drinking at least 3.5 ounces of liquid every five minutes (approximately every kilometer) of their run. This requires practice. If it is hot, throwing cold water over your body is fine. It can help bring down your core body temperature.

COME RAIN OR SHINE

Weather is the one element you cannot control on race day. It often catches racers off guard. Few of us probably visualize the potential weather condition of race days. If you race often enough, you are bound to have an extremely hot or cold day once in a while.

Racing attire can dramatically improve the comfort of racing in less than ideal conditions. Wetsuits and neoprene swim caps make cold swims bearable, waterproof breathable rain gear can stave off the biting cold on wet and windy rides, and a hat can keep the scorching sun off your face and head. Also, Vaseline™ can help to reduce chafing in the swim, cycle and on the run.

The colors you wear should also complement the weather. If it is sunny and hot, wear lighter clothing. If it is cold, wear darker colors. Layered clothing can also be advantageous. If it starts to warm up you can always take off layers.

You have a choice: you can either be properly prepared and give it your best, or simply choose not to race, but, do not use the weather as an excuse for a dismal performance. All the other contenders have to deal with the same conditions. The satisfaction of completing a race under such circumstances can be exhilarating. Be flexible. Life will go on even if you don't do as well as you wanted and, in years to come, what will it matter? If you can keep your spirits high during these times, the weather will almost always work to your advantage. It is your health and fitness that counts, not the race.

MASTERING THE POST-RACE

In 1978 I. Dragan, a Romanian scientist, studied the recovery of athletes in the twenty-four hours after competition. He found that heart rate and blood pressure recover in twenty to sixty minutes following strenuous effort; restoration of glucosides takes four to six hours; protein restoration takes twelve to twenty-four hours; and fats, vitamins and enzymes take over twenty-four hours to recover. Recovery time, however, depends on many things including:

▸ *Age.* The younger you are the faster you recover.

▸ *Experience.* The more experience you have training and racing, the less time you'll need to recover.

▸ *Gender.* Women typically take longer to recover than men.

▸ *Environment.* Factors such as altitude, time zone changes and humidity play a role in recovery rates.

Researchers have shown that recovery varies from person to person. One of the first things you need to do after a race is properly cool down. It is usually a good idea to go for a walk, an easy jog or ride twenty to thirty minutes after the race to help your system eliminate the lactic acid build-up. Swimming is also fine. The short rest will allow your body to recover from the physical exertion. It will also give you some time to ingest needed fluids and nutrients.

If you decide to get a massage, wait fifteen to twenty minutes before jumping on the table otherwise your muscles may tighten up and the actual massage may be quite painful. Most good therapists will ask you how long it has been since you finished racing. Your body needs to cool down naturally before you begin to manipulate it. A good massage is almost like another workout.

Post-event feeding is also critical to the recovery process. The first ten hours after a race (or hard training) are the most important for recovery. After the race, stay away from those tempting cookies, sodas and alcoholic drinks which are often available. These provide either empty calories or only simple sugars, neither of which will replenish the complex carbohydrates and electrolytes your body needs. Remember, no matter how fit you are or how often you've raced, you need to treat your body well if you want it to continue to perform for you! Focus on consuming water (preferably distilled), vegetable soup and wholewheat products such as fig bars and bagels.

RECOVERY

For a day or two after a hard race, do not try any strenuous workouts. Listen to your body and allow it to recover properly. Try to avoid running, regardless of how good you feel! Walking is a great means of recovery and allows you to stretch your legs. If time permits, I will usually go for a good walk the evening after a race.

Consider trying several natural means of assisting your recovery. These range from kinotherapy (in which you lightly exercise muscle groups other than those used in the race), extra sleep, massage, reflexology, ultrasound or electrostimulation of sore muscles, and even oxygen therapy. Practice and experiment with what works best for you but don't be afraid to try new things in the off-season. Keep a log of what works best and monitor your heart rate and pH levels.

Develop a ritual so that nothing is unexpected. This may be why so many athletes have superstitions – if something works for them they stick with it.

DOING YOUR BEST IS REALLY ALL THAT MATTERS

Be realistic about your goals and objectives. Know your pace and your limits. This is what you have trained for. And while unforeseen incidents may happen, they are all part of racing and life. The more you know of yourself the easier it will be to have fun and keep a healthy and active lifestyle.

Over the years, some coaches have made their mark based on their hard-nosed attitude that winning was all that counts. No one remembers who finished second! Well, when it comes to sponsors and race promotion, this is probably true. Until Mark Allen finally won the Hawaii Ironman (after six losses), his top ten finishes meant little more than making the "good chance" list.

Racing is about winning within yourself and *knowing you did your best*. As long as you have trained properly and know your limits, gauge your success against what you know you are capable of. March to the beat of your own drum. If at the end of the day you can say you feel good about your performance, then you are a winner. As the Olympic oath says, "Let me win, but if I cannot win, let me be brave in the attempt."

CONCLUSION

We trust that you have found this book informative and entertaining and that you will want to refer to it from time to time to brush up on important points or simply to re-inspire yourself.

Remember that while this book may inspire you to adopt a more active and healthy lifestyle, it is up to you to maintain this for the rest of your life! As you age and take on new responsibilities, your health and fitness priorities may change. Life is full of wonderful opportunities and you should experience them to the fullest.

Appendix: Fitness Level Tests

The following fitness tests are considered fairly standard in most university and college physical education based programs. So if you would rather have someone help you, check with your local university or college about getting tested in your flexibility, overall fitness, endurance and strength. Most of these tests are adapted from H.B. Falls, A.M. Baylor and R.K. Dishman's book, *Essentials of Fitness.**

FLEXIBILITY

1. Lay down flat on your chest and extend your back to see how far you can lift your neck from the floor. Have someone measure the distance from the floor to your sternal notch (where your chin meets your neck). This is measurement *a*.

2. Sitting with your back and buttocks against a wall, measure the distance from the floor to your sternal notch. This is measurement *b*.

3. Your flexibility score can be calculated as:

$$\frac{a \times 100}{b}$$

Rating:

Less than 25: very poor   25–35: poor
36–45: average   46–50: good
51–55: very good   56–57: excellent
58+: superior

STRENGTH RATING

Strength tests require you test four different muscle groups. Here you want to determine the maximum weight you can lift

---

* *Essentials of Fitness* © 1980 by H.B. Falls, A.M. Baylor and R.K. Dishman. New York: McGraw-Hill. Reproduced with the permission of the McGraw-Hill Companies.

in one rep only. Start with a weight you feel is close to your maximum and then add weight until you can complete the lift *once*. Remember to do a proper warm-up before you begin this test.

1) (a) bench press with wide grip

   (b) leg press

   (c) bicep curl (free weight bar)

   (d) shoulder press (free weight bar)

2) Divide the amount of weight lifted in each test by your present body weight to determine the percent of weight lifted. You can then apply this figure to the Strength Rating Chart in order to measure yourself against others.

Table A1 STRENGTH RATING CHART (MALE/FEMALE)

% weight lifted	Poor	Low	Average	Good	Very Good	Excellent
bench press	50/40	75/60	100/70	110/75	120/80	140+/90+
leg press	160/100	180/120	200/140	210/145	220/150	230+/175+
bicep curl	30/15	40/20	50/35	55/40	60/45	70+/55+
shoulder press	40/20	50/30	67/47	70/55	80/60	110+/60+

ENDURANCE RATING

A wide variety of endurance tests exist. Rather than present them all here, I will include one of the most common tests – push-ups. If you are interested in expanding your endurance-testing repertoire, seek out a good general fitness book. For example, there are post-exercise pulse count fitness charts; swim, cycling and two-minute jogging tests; and even do-it-yourself body fat charts.

PUSH-UPS

Men should use the standard push-up position with legs fully extended and your body supported by your toes and hands. Women should use the modified push-up, i.e., begin with knees touching the floor instead of trying to support all your weight with your hands and toes. Count the number of consecutive push-ups you can do. Be sure to bring your chest to the floor or fist-distance from the floor (an assistant can help here). Take your score and compare to the following table to find your endurance level.

Table A2 ENDURANCE RATING (MALE/FEMALE)

Age	Poor	Low	Average	Good	Very Good	Excellent
15–29	<19/<5	<25/<9	<34/<16	<44/<33	<50/<45	>54/>48
30–39	<14/<3	<20/<7	<24/<11	<40/<24	<40/<33	>44/>37
40–49	<11/<2	<14/<5	<19/<7	<29/<19	<35/<28	>39/>32
50–59	<7/<1	<12/<3	<14/<5	<24/<14	<30/<21	>34/>25
60–69	<4/<1	<7/<2	<9/<3	<19/<4	<25/<15	>29/>19

These three tests will indicate your overall fitness level. Now assess whether the total number of hours you spent training and racing last year fairly matches the effort you put into the sport. For example, if your focus is primarily short course events, and assuming you trained around three hundred hours – an average of about 6.25 hours per week, you should be above average in all-round fitness. If not, you can assume you are either overtraining or training inappropriately and you should adjust your regimen accordingly. You should also consider whether you are properly balancing your aerobic and anaerobic workouts – they should be about eighty percent aerobic and twenty percent anaerobic. If, however, you do find yourself in good to excellent shape for the time you spend training, then Table A3 below will recommend how much you should increase your volume of training in the coming year.

If you trained less than two hundred hours last year then, depending on your level of fitness, you can increase your next year's volume by three to eight percent. If you are already training between 800 and 900 hours a year (about fourteen hours per week) you should only increase your next year's volume by five percent. Needless to say, most of us do not have the time to train more than fourteen hours per week (two hours a day) and, fortunately, you do not need to in order to maintain a healthy and active lifestyle. Only if you are training competitively for an Ironman distance race is there any rationale to do over 500 hours a year. Should you already be at that level then your criterion performances (discussed in Chapter 12) and monitoring become even more vital – you should be able to get by on less if you follow the criterion tests and TRIMPS program!

Table A3 PERCENTAGE INCREASE IN YEARLY TRAINING HOURS

HOURS	PERCEIVED LEVEL OF FITNESS				
	Poor	Low	Average	Good	Excellent
<200	3%	4%	5–6%	7%	8%
201–300		4%	6–7%	7%	8%
301–400			7–8%	8–9%	10%
401–500			8%	10%	12%
501–600			10%	12%	14%
601–700				13–14%	14%
701–800				10%	10%
801–900				5%	5%

Glossary

ABSORPTION – the process by which nutrients enter the bloodstream through the digestive system.

ACID-ALKALINE BALANCE – see pH.

ADAPTOGEN – a supplement, herb or food that increases the body's ability to cope with physical, emotional, chemical and biological stress.

ADENOSINE TRIPHOSPHATE (ATP) – one of the four most important energy-containing chemical elements in the body. It is the only element that can supply energy for muscle contraction. When depleted, the body "runs out of steam" and slows down.

AEROBIC – describes a process or activity that requires the use of oxygen.

AEROBIC WORKOUT – an activity that raises the heart rate to at least sixty percent of its maximum.

AFFIRMATION – a positive statement or phrase that strengthens and focuses the mind.

AMINO ACID – any one of over twenty compounds that form the building blocks of protein in the body. Each amino acid performs specific functions. They are made by the body or can be supplied in the diet.

ANABOLIC STEROID – a synthetic variation of the male hormone testosterone which provides shortcuts to improved performance, strength and muscle mass. Steroids are illegal in competitive sport and can be deadly (see Chapter 14).

ANAEROBIC – describes an activity or process that does not require the use of oxygen.

ANAEROBIC WORKOUT – an activity that raises the heart rate to seventy-five percent or more of its maximum. This is a stress-inducing activity that also improves speed and strength.

ANEMIA (SPORTS) – a condition in which one has below normal hemoglobin levels or low iron counts. Many endurance athletes are prone to anemia so careful blood monitoring is essential in these cases. Runners may be especially susceptible to iron loss through bleeding of minute blood vessels in the soles of the feet; this is known as footstrike hematosis or runner's hematosis.

ANTIOXIDANT – a compound that reacts with and neutralizes unpaired oxygen molecules to protect other compounds from oxidation. Antioxidants, usually vitamins, minerals or enzymes, protect the body from free radical attacks.

ASSIMILATION – a process that occurs when food is absorbed and its nutrients are used constructively by the body.

ATHLETE – a person who participates in exercise, games or sports requiring a degree of physical agility, endurance and strength.

ATP – see adenosine triphosphate.

BODY FAT – refers to the percent of fat tissue in the body. Most experts agree that healthy males should have no more than twenty-three percent body fat while healthy women should have no more than twenty-seven percent body fat. Women need more body fat to meet the energy needs of menstruation, pregnancy and breastfeeding. Body fat among athletes will vary depending on the sport.

BOWEL TOLERANCE – the highest level of a particular substance (usually vitamin C) you can take without causing diarrhea.

CARBOHYDRATE – one of the three major sources of energy in food. There are simple and complex carbohydrates. Simple carbohydrates contain simple sugars and provide short-term energy. Complex carbohydrates are necessary for athletes and others who want a sustained level of energy.

CARCINOGEN – any product that causes cancer.

CHOLESTEROL – a fatty substance that has many vital functions in the body. Cholesterol is found naturally in the brain, nerves, liver, blood and bile, and is supplied by consuming animal foods. "Good" cholesterol is HDL cholesterol and "bad" cholesterol is LDL cholesterol.

CLEANSING – the process of naturally eliminating toxins from the body using a series of steps which includes eating fresh fruits and vegetables, fasting with juices and taking homeopathic remedies.

COOL-DOWN – a necessary step after heavy training or racing. Cooling down allows the body to recover and helps you to eliminate lactic acid build-up. It is also a time to take in needed fluids and nutrients. A cool down may involve a walk, an easy jog, a short ride or an easy swim.

CROSS TRAINING – participating in a variety of athletic activities that have a beneficial effect on other (physical) activities. For example, cross-country skiing has excellent aerobic benefits which will improve your ability to cycle, run and swim.

ELECTROLYTE – a mineral salt in the body that influences muscular action and oxygen consumption. The most common electrolyte is sodium.

ENDURANCE – building a strong aerobic base that allows you to participate in an activity for a long period of time without fatiguing.

ENERGY – the capacity for activity. Many elements in food are transformed and stored as energy in the body. Also, the body is comprised of a complex network of energy fields which, in Chinese medicine is called the vital force, or *chi*.

ERGOGENIC – a substance that enhances performance. Controversial products involve anabolic steroids (Chapter 14) while natural alternatives include a wide range of other herbs and supplements.

EXERCISE – an activity requiring physical effort.

FAT (DIETARY) – the body's most concentrated source of energy.

FATTY ACIDS – the main building blocks of fats and oils. Fatty acids are important for providing energy and they play key roles in the function of all cells and tissues. Fatty acids are supplied by food and they are generated by the body as well. Essential fatty acids cannot be made by the body and must be supplied in the diet. The two essential fatty acids are the omega-3 alpha-linolenic acid and omega-6 linoleic acid.

FEAR – a physiological reaction to an event or situation that can interfere with clear thinking and undermine self-confidence and performance.

FITNESS – the physical ability to perform a particular athletic activity.

FLEXIBILITY – the ability of a joint to move through its full range of motion. Poor flexibility is usually due to muscle tightness – a common cause of stress-related injuries.

FREE RADICAL – a highly reactive compound in the body which, in excessive amounts, can cause cell damage. Free radicals are produced by normal body metabolism and by factors such as exposure to radiation and environmental pollutants. Damage from free radicals is linked to aging, cancer, immune system impairment and heart disease.

GEAR – a set of toothed wheels on a bicycle that are used in different combinations for speed and power. Also commonly refers to clothing and equipment. Goggles and wetsuits are examples of swimming gear.

GLYCOGEN – the stored form of glucose that is used by cells for energy.

HEALTH – a state of well-being in the mind and body. Health is determined by many factors such as socioeconomic conditions, culture and environment.

HEART RATE TARGET ZONE – indicates the intensity at which you should work out. You should calculate your upper and lower heart rate limits for effective training (see Chapter 12).

HOLISM – a healing approach that treats the whole person: the body, mind, and spirit as well as social, economic, hereditary and environmental factors.

Holism centers on the healing power of nature, the responsibility of the patient in recovery and the maintenance of good health; it places emphasis on prevention, a healthy lifestyle and the use of natural substances to strengthen the body.

HOMEOPATHY – a non-toxic system of medicine used to treat a wide variety of illnesses. Founded by the German physician Samuel Hahnemann, the formulations are based on three principles: 1) like cures like, 2) the more a remedy is diluted the greater its potency, and 3) an illness is specific to the individual. Therefore, each case must be treated separately.

HOMEOSTASIS – the tendency toward stability in the body's interdependent systems.

INFLAMMATION – the immune system's reaction to injury or irritation, usually characterized by heat, pain, redness or swelling.

INTERVAL – a type of workout that helps build speed and strength. It involves high-intensity bursts followed by a recovery period.

LACTIC ACID – a substance that builds up when the muscles are depleted of glycogen (e.g., from exercise). Muscles become sore, movement becomes inefficient and cramping may also occur.

LIPIDS – a collective term for any fatty substance, including fats, oils, steroids and fatty acids. (See also Fat.)

MAXIMUM AEROBIC PACE (MAP) – (defined by Phillip Maffetone) the aerobic heart rate at which people should spend approximately eighty percent of their training time. As the body adapts to performing a certain distance at a fixed aerobic heart rate, distance traveled can then be increased while maintaining same heart rate.

METABOLISM – the total of all chemical and physical processes in the body that convert nutritive material into living matter and energy.

MINERAL – any of the twenty elements necessary for a healthy body that must be supplied by the diet. Minerals act with enzymes, vitamins, hormones and other substances in many functions. Calcium and sodium are common major minerals. *Trace minerals*, such as chromium and zinc, are required by the body in small amounts.

MOTIVATION – ideas or objects that stimulate individual interest in an activity.

NATUROPATHIC MEDICINE – a distinct system of primary health care that uses natural methods and substances to support and stimulate the body's self-healing ability.

NUTRITION – the sum of the processes involved in assimilating nutrients from food to sustain life, provide energy and maintain health.

OMEGA-3 FATTY ACIDS – a family of fatty acids derived from the essential alpha-linolenic acid. Included in this family is eicosapentaenoic acid (EPA), which occurs naturally in the body and in fish oils.

OMEGA-6 FATTY ACIDS – a family of fatty acids derived from the essential linoleic acid.

OPTIMAL HEALTH – a state of mind, body and spirit that allows for optimal function.

PEAKING – the point where physical and mental training enables you to perform at your full potential during a race.

PERIODIZATION – a form of training where the type and amount of training is varied and divided into phases or periods (See Chapter 4).

pH – a measure of acidity or alkalinity of a substance. The pH scale runs from zero to fourteen; a pH of seven is neutral, less than seven is acidic, and over seven is alkaline. In the body, pH balance, commonly called the acid-alkaline balance, is regulated by the body's fluids and electrolytes.

PROTEIN – the body's second most plentiful substance; it is essential for proper growth and development. It is the major building block for muscle, blood, hair, internal organs and nails. Protein also plays an essential role in the formation of various growth hormones and determines your rate of metabolism. Stress, or hard exercise, can deplete the body of protein. It should then be replenished in order to stay fit and healthy.

PRECURSOR – a parent substance that must be present before another substance, usually a vitamin, is manufactured by the body or by cooking. For example, beta-carotene is a precursor to vitamin A in the body.

RESISTANCE EXERCISE – an exercise that subjects the muscles to repeated and progressive resistance. This increases the muscle's ability to perform more efficiently since it increases both strength and endurance.

RESTORATION – resting the body after the racing season by participating in low-intensity activities such as hot showers or baths, saunas, massage, relaxation and stretching, and vitamin and mineral build-up.

RITUALS – the consistent effort and practice of routines and/or activities.

SPEED – an ability to perform an activity quickly and at a high anaerobic level.

STAMINA – the ability to perform with intensity over a long period.

STRENGTH TRAINING – weight training to build strength.

STRESS – a physical, chemical, thermal and emotional state that interferes with the body's ability to adapt to emotional and physical demands.

STRETCHING – exercises designed to prepare the body for a more strenuous workout. Stretching increases flexibility, relaxes muscles, increases blood flow, creates awareness of body motions and decreases the likelihood of injury.

SUPPLEMENT – a substance that provides nutrients, such as vitamins and minerals, to maintain health, to prevent or treat illness and to compensate for dietary deficiencies. Athletes often take supplements to provide for high nutritional needs.

SYNERGY – the interaction of two or more substances which together create a stronger effect than the effect of each individual substance.

TAPERING – reducing the intensity and duration of workouts. It is usually done prior to racing to build energy reserves.

TEMPO – a continuous effort lasting 20–30 minutes with your heart rate in your anaerobic threshold. (Your heart rate could rise five beats above or below your anaerobic threshold.)

TOXIN – a poison. Any substance that impairs the proper functioning of the body. Natural toxins are produced by living organisms; unnatural toxins such as pesticides, additives and pollutants contaminate our food supply.

TRAINING IMPULSE SCORE (TRIMPS) – a measurement combining your heart rate and the duration of an activity to determine the quality of a workout and to get the best results from your training. This measurement can also help you reduce the risk of overtraining and prevent injury.

TRANSITION – the changeover in a multidisciplinary race from one sport to another, such as swim-to-bike transition or bike-to-run transition. The need to save seconds, especially in short races, has resulted in the transition becoming almost a science.

TRIATHLON – an athletic event involving three separate sporting activities. The traditional combination involves swimming, cycling and running. Seasonal variations (e.g., snowshoeing, cross-country skiing and ice speed skating) also occur. Distances for the individual sections vary with the "Olympic distance" having a .93 mile (1.5 km) swim, a 24.8 mile (40 km) cycle, and a 6.2 mile (10 km) run.

TRIMPS – see Training Impulse Score.

VISUALIZATION (SPORTS) – relaxation exercises involving positive mental images of a desired goal.

VITAMIN – any of the thirteen nutrients essential for the body that must be obtained from the diet. Different vitamins regulate metabolic processes and are important antioxidants. Vitamins are lost in processed foods.

WARM-UP – exercises performed before hard physical activity to relieve tension, raise the heart rate slightly and to work up a light sweat. A warm-up may involve a short jog with wind sprints, a five to ten minute ride on a stationary trainer or a short swim.

WEIGHT TRAINING – using weights to build strength and endurance.

Bibliography

Anderson, O. 1995, April. "The Fast Lane: Precision Training." *Runner's World:* 36.

Bahna, S.L. and D.C. Henier. 1980. *Allergies to Milk.* New York: Grune and Stratton.

Bailey, C. 1991. *The New Fit or Fat.* Boston: Houghton Mifflin.

Balch, James F. and Phyllis A. Balch. 1997. *Prescription for Natural Healing.* Garden City Park, NY: Avery Publishing.

Beasley, J.A. and J.J. Swift. 1989. *The Kellogg Report.* Annandale-on-Hudson, NY: Institute of Health Policy and Practice, Bard College Center.

Becker, G. 1997. *The Gift of Fear.* Boston: Little Brown.

Burke, E. 1986. *Science of Cycling.* Champaign, IL: Human Kinetic Book.

Burton Goldberg Group. 1994. *Alternative Medicine: The Definitive Guide.* Puyallup, WA: Future Medicine.

Calbom, C. and M. Keane. 1992. *Juicing for Life.* Salt Lake City, UT: Publishers Press.

California Department of Consumer Affairs (CDCA). 1982. "Clean Your Room: A Compendium of Indoor Pollution." Sacramento, CA: State of California.

Canadian Fitness and Lifestyle Research. 1988. Ottawa: Canadian Fitness and Lifestyle Institute.

Chopra, D. 1989. *Quantum Healing.* New York: Bantam Books.

———. 1990. *Perfect Health.* New York: Bantam Books.

———. 1993. *Ageless Body, Timeless Mind.* New York: Harmony Books.

———. 1994. *Restful Sleep.* New York: Bantam Books.

Clohessy, P. 1995, June. "Training for the Veteran Long Distance Runner." *The Masters Athlete:* 6.

Colgan, M. 1993. *Optimum Sports Nutrition: Your Competitive Edge.* New York: Advanced Research Press.

———. 1994. *The New Nutrition: Medicine for the Millenium.* San Diego, CA: C.I. Publications.

Cook, B. and G. Stewart. 1996. *Strength Basics: Your Guide to Resistance Training for Health and Optimal Performance.* Champaign, IL: Human Kinetic Book.

Csikszentmihalyi. 1988. *Optimal Experience*. Cambridge University Press.

D'Adamo, J. 1989. *The D'Adamo Diet*. Toronto: McGraw-Hill.

D'Adamo, P.J. 1996. *Eat Right 4 Your Type*. New York: Putnam.

Diamond, M. 1987. *A New Way of Eating*. New York: Warner Books.

Falls, H.B., A.M. Baylor and R.K. Dishman. 1980. *Essentials of Fitness*. Philadelphia, PA: Sander College; Holt, Rinehart, and Winston.

Douillard, J. 1991. *Invincible Athletics*. Lancaster, MA: Maharishi Ayur-Veda.

Dragam AM, et al. 1987. "Studies Concerning the Ergogenic Value of Protein Supply and L-carnitine in Elite Athletes." *Physiologie* 24: 231–234 [1987].

Edwards, S. 1994, Jan./Feb. "Basic Training Using a Heart Monitor." *Triathlete*: 22–23.

Erasmus, U. 1993. *Fats that Heal Fats that Kill*. Burnaby, BC: *alive* books.

Erickson, E. 1978. *Adulthood*. New York: Norton.

Foot, D. and Daniel Stoffman 1996. *Boom, Bust and Echo*. Toronto: Macfarlane Walter and Ross.

Force, J. 1997, May 15. *Concept Mapping Workshop*. Nakoda Lodge, AB. (presentation).

Galloway, J. 1984. *Galloway's Book on Running*. Bolinas, CA: Shelter Pub.

Garfield, C.A. 1984. *Peak Performance*. Boston: Houghton Mifflin.

Garrison, Robert and Elizabeth Somer. 1995. *The Nutrition Desk Reference*. New Canaan, CT: Keats Publishing.

Gerber, Richard. 1988. *Vibrational Medicine*. Santa Fe, NM: Bear & Company.

Graci, S. 1997. *The Power of Superfoods*. Scarborough, ON: Prentice-Hall.

Gursche, S. 1993. *Healing with Herbal Juices*. Burnaby, BC: *alive* books.

Haas, R. 1983. *Eat to Win*. New York: New American Library.

Habib, M. 1996, Sept. 9. "Resistance Training: It's More Than Just Pumping Iron." *Calgary Herald*: B8.

Hamilton, K. and H. Trepanier. 1994. "Hospital Care in the 21st Century." *Canadian Social Trends: A Canadian Studies Reader*. Vol. 2. Toronto: Thompson Educational Publication: 95–98.

Hay, L.L. 1984. *You Can Heal Your Life*. Santa Monica, CA: Hay House.

———. 1988. *Heal Your Body*. Santa Monica, CA: Hay House.

Heider, J. 1986. *The Tao of Leadership*. New York: Bantam.

Henderson, J. (Ed.). 1978. *The Runner's Diet*. Mountain View, CA: World Pub.

Heuts, Oliver. 1997. *It's Never Too Late to Look and Feel Younger Through Exercise*, Pilot Books.

Hoff, B. 1982. *The Tao of Pooh*. New York: Viking Penguin.

Howard, J. 1992, Dec./Jan. "Bike fit." *Velo News*: 43–46.

———. 1993, October. "Crank it Up." *Triathlete*: 12.

Hoy. Claire. 1995. *The Truth About Breast Cancer*. Toronto: Stoddart.

JAMA. 1994. Vol. 1.

Janssen, Peter. 1987. *Training, Lactate, Pulse Rate*. Oy Liitto, Finland: Polar Electro Oy.

Lanctot, G. 1995. *The Medical Mafia*. Miami: Here's the Key Inc.

Lancet. 1993, Oct. 23. Vol. 342.

Lavinson, D. and K. Christensen, (Eds.). 1996. *World Sports III*. Santa Barbara, CA: ABC-Clio.

LeMond, G. and K. Gordis. 1987. *The Complete Book of Cycling*. New York: The Putnam Publishing Group.

Lewis, N. 1998, Jan. "Bagels Effective as Energy Food." *Calgary Herald*: D6.

Loehr, J.E. and P.J. McLaughlin. 1986. *Mentally Tough*. New York: M. Evans and Co.

Lynch, J. 1987. *The Total Runner*. Englewood Cliffs, NJ: Prentice-Hall.

Lynch, J.M. 1992, May. "The Deal with Wheels." *Triathlete*: 46–52.

Maffetone, P. 1989. *Everyone is an Athlete*. Stamford, NY: David Barmore Productions.

———. 1997. *In Fitness and In Health*. 3rd edition. New York: David Barmore Productions.

Maglischo, E.W. 1988. *Swimming Faster*. Mountain View, CA: Mayfield.

———. 1993. *Swimming Even Faster*. Mountain View, CA: Mayfield.

Moore, T. 1994. *Soul Mates*. New York: HarperCollins.

Morton, R.H., J. Fitz-Clarke and E.W. Banister. 1990. "Modeling human performance in running." *Journal of Applied Physiology* 69: 1171–1177.

Murphy, M. 1993. *The Future of the Body*. New York: Jeremy P. Tarcher/Perigee Books.

National Research Council. 1989. *Diet and Health: Implications for Reducing Chronic Disease Risk*. Washington: National Academy Press.

Olinekova, G. 1988. *Winning Without Steroids*. New Canaan, CT: Keats.

Oski, F. 1992. *Don't Drink Your Milk*. Brushton, NY: Teach Services.

Pearl, B. and G.T. Moran. 1986. *Getting Stronger*. Bolinas, CA: Shelter.

Pearson, D. and S. Shaw. 1983. *Life Extension: Weight Loss Program*. New York: Doubleday.

Pitchford, P. 1993. *Healing With Whole Foods*. Berkeley, CA: North Atlantic Books.

Reaburn, P. 1995, June. "Interval Training for Older Athletes." *The Masters Athlete*: 1.

———. 1995, June. "Get Strong – Get Fast." *The Masters Athlete*: 9.

Reddan, G. 1995, June. "Strength Training for Triathlon." *The Masters Athlete*: 11.

Robbins, A. 1986. *Unlimited Power*. New York: Fawcett Columbine.

Schauss, A. 1980. *Diet, Crime and Delinquency*. Berkeley, CA: Parker House.

Sears, B. 1995. *Enter the Zone*. New York: Harper and Row.

Selye, H. 1956. *The Stress of Life*. New York: McGraw-Hill.

———. 1974. *Stress Without Distress*. New York: New American Library.

Shealy, N. 1996. *The Complete Family Guide to Alternative Medicine*. Rockport, MA: Element Books.

Sheehan, G. 1992, June. "New Fitness Formula." *Runner's World*: 18.

Sheehy, G. 1995. *New Passages*. New York: Random House.

Shepley, B. 1992. "Personal Best: Triathlon Training Seminar." Calgary, AB.

Sisco, Peter and John Little. 1997. *Power Factor Training*. Boise, ID: Power Factor Publishing Inc.

Sisson, M. 1989. *Training and Racing Biathlons*. Los Angeles: Primal Urge Press.

Sleamaker, R. and Ray Browning. 1989. *Serious Training for Endurance Athletes*. Champaign, IL: Leisure Press.

Souza, Ken. 1989. *Biathalon: Training and Racing Techniques*. Chicago, IL: Contemporary Books.

Stewart, G. 1980. *Every Body's Fitness Book*. New York: A Dolphin Book.

Subotnick, S. 1991. *Sports and Exercise Injury*. Berkeley, CA: North Atlantic Books.

Thompson, P. and C. Bird. 1992. *The Secret Life of Plants*. New York: Harper and Row.

Tobias, M. and J.P. Sullivan. 1992. *Complete Stretching: A New Exercise Program for Health and Vitality*. Toronto: Random House.

Townsend Letter. 1995, Feb./March.

Treben, M. 1987. *Health from God's Garden*. Rochester, VT: Thorsons.

Turner, C.V. 1996. "The Five-Step Conversion." *Triathlete*: 66–69.

Whitaker, J. 1995, Jan. *Health and Healing.* (Newsletter).

Wiley, R. 1989. *Biobalancing.* Tacoma, WA: Life Science Press.

Williams, M.H. 1989. *Beyond Training: How Athletes Enhance Performance Legally and Illegally.* Champaign, IL: Leisure Press.

Winterdyk, J. 1992. "Triathlete Profile Survey." *Transition.* 1(3): 7–8.

Wintrop-Young, G. 1977. *Book of Selected Readings.* South River, ON: Project DARE.

Zempel, C. 1992, Nov. "Bubble Hand, Breathe Hand: Time to Tackle Bilateral Breathing." *Triathlete*: 18–19.

Copyright Acknowledgments

COPYRIGHT ACKNOWLEDGEMENTS

Every reasonable attempt was made to contact Dr. Karvonen for permission to reprint his Training Heart Rate Calculation.

Janssen's Heart Rate Calculation was drawn from his book *Training, Lactate, Pulse Rate* published by Polar Electro Oy of Finland. Every reasonable attempt was made to contact Peter Janssen for permission to reprint his material.

Léger's Heart Rate Calculation and the information in Table 12.2 on heart rates for cycling and running are reprinted with the permission of Dr. Luc Léger of the University of Montréal.

Maffetone's Heart Rate Calculation and the Maximum Aerobic Pace (MAP) is excerpted with the permission of Philip Maffetone from *In Fitness and In Health*. Copyrighted © 1997 by Philip Maffetone and published by David Barmore Productions, Stamford, NY.

The Training Impulse Score (TRIMPS) program is excerpted and adapted with the permission of the publisher from *Journal of Applied Physiology*, "Modeling Human Performance in Running," (1990, 69: 1171–1177) by R.H. Morton, J. Fitz-Clarke and E.W. Banister. Published by The American Physiological Society, Bethesda, MD.

The quote from Owen Anderson is reprinted by permission of *Runner's World Magazine*. Copyrighted 1995. Rodale Press, Inc., all rights reserved.

The chart, Common Problems and Probable Causes, from *Heal Your Body* by Louise Hay, is used by permission of Hay House, Inc., Carlsbad, CA.

The Yin and Yang chart is reprinted from *Alternative Medicine: The Definitive Guide*, p. 452 with permission by Future Medicine Publishing, Inc., 21-1/2 Main Street, Tiburon, CA 94920 (800) 333-HEAL.

Table 15.1 Effects of Exercise Layoff is adapted from *Galloway's Book on Running*, © 1984 by Jeff Galloway. $13.00. Shelter Publications, Inc., P.O. Box 279, Bolinas, CA 94924. Distributed in bookstores by Random House. Reprinted by permission.

Training recommendations by Gale Bernhardt are reprinted by permission of *Triathlete* magazine.

Table A3 Percent Increase in Yearly Training Hours is adapted by permission from R. Sleamaker and R. Browning 1989, *Serious Training for Endurance Athletes* (Champaign, IL: Human Kinetics), 24.

Index

Date Due